Research Design and Analysis

Mention of specific products or equipment by contributors to this AABB Press publication does not represent an endorsement of such products by the AABB Press nor does it necessarily indicate a preference for those products over other similar competitive products.

Efforts are made to have publications of the AABB Press consistent in regard to acceptable practices. However, for several reasons, they may not be. First, as new developments in the practice of blood banking occur, changes may be recommended to the AABB *Standards for Blood Banks and Transfusion Services.* It is not possible, however, to revise each publication at the time such a change is adopted. Thus, it is essential that the most recent edition of the *Standards* be consulted as a reference in regard to current acceptable practices. Second, the views expressed in this publication represent the opinions of the authors. The publication of this book does not constitute an endorsement by the AABB Press of any view expressed herein, and the AABB Press expressly disclaims any liability arising from any inaccuracy or misstatement.

Research Design and Analysis

Editors

Mark E. Brecher, MD
Director, Transplantation and Transfusion Services
Department of Hospital Laboratories
University of North Carolina Hospitals
University of North Carolina—Chapel Hill
Transfusion Medicine
Chapel Hill, North Carolina

Michael P. Busch, MD, PhD
Vice President, Research and Science Services
Blood Centers of the Pacific-Irwin Center
Professor of Laboratory Medicine
University of California, San Francisco
San Francisco, California

American Association of Blood Banks
Bethesda, Maryland
1998

Copyright © 1998 by the American Association of Blood Banks. All rights reserved. Reproduction or transmission of text in any form or by any means, electronic or mechanical, including photocopying, recording, or by any information storage and retrieval system is prohibited without permission in writing from the Publisher.

The Publisher has made every effort to trace the copyright holders for borrowed material. If they have inadvertently overlooked any, they will be pleased to make the necessary arrangements at the first opportunity.

American Association of Blood Banks
8101 Glenbrook Road
Bethesda, Maryland 20814-2749

ISBN NO. 1-56395-100-2
Printed in the United States

Contents

Foreword ix

1. Primary Study Design 1

James J. Korelitz, PhD, and D. Robert Harris, PhD

General Categories of Study Designs 2
Specific Types of Study Designs 3
Study Designs Applied to Issues in Blood
    Banking and Transfusion Medicine 6
Planning and Conducting Studies 20
Summary 25
References 26

2. Meta-Analysis and Study Design 31

*Eleftherios C. Vamvakas, MD, MPhil, PhD,
MPH, MPA*

The Use of Meta-Analysis 32
Component Parts of a Meta-Analysis 35
Rationale for Restricting Meta-Analyses to
    Randomized Controlled Trials 39
Assessment of the Quality of Randomized
    Controlled Trials for Inclusion in a
    Meta-Analysis 46
Conclusion 54
References 55

3. Statistical Analysis 63

Michael H. Kanter, MD

Statistical Analysis as a Type of Mathematical
    Model 64
The Importance of p Values in Medical Research . . 65

Use of Confidence Intervals Instead of p Values—
A Solution to the Limitations of p Values 87
p Values Cannot Be Used to Compare the Baseline
Characteristics of Randomized Groups 89
Descriptive Statistics 91
Summary. 98
References 98

4. **Human Subjects Research in the Blood Banking Environment: Institutional Review Board Approval and Informed Consent. . . 105**

   Judith A. Hautala, PhD

   Background 106
   Criteria for IRB Review and Approval 109
   Impact of Human Subjects Research Regulations
   on Study Design. 113
   Informed Consent 117
   Facilitating the IRB Review Process 122
   Human Subjects Research Issues Relevant to
   Blood Banking 124
   Conclusion 129
   References 130

5. **The Publication of Research Results. . . . 131**

   Jeffrey McCullough, MD

   Planning the Research Project 131
   Disseminating the Results. 137
   Conclusions 147

6. **NHLBI Support for Biomedical Research and Training. 149**

   George J. Nemo, PhD

   Program Overview 149
   Investigator-Initiated Research 151

Institute-Initiated Research Programs: The Process
 of Planning, Developing, and Implementing
 Initiatives 152
Distribution of the Division of Blood Diseases and
Resources Budget by Funding Mechanism 154
Transfusion Medicine Scientific Research Group:
 Current Institute-Initiated Research Activities. . 157
Types of Grant Mechanisms 161
Grants to Support Research Career
 Development 165
National Research Service Awards (NRSA) 167
Minority Programs. 168
Summary 170

Index **171**

Foreword

These presentations from the program "Research Design and Analysis" form an overdue follow-up to a previously successful workshop entitled "Successful Research Design and Publication." The future of our field is dependent on cultivating a new generation of researchers and supporting those researchers currently in the field. We are particularly cognizant of the frequent perception by novices that initiating a successful research program is an overwhelming undertaking.

For perspective, one can think of science as a moving train constantly and inexorably moving forward. As a student or novice researcher, one must run to catch that moving train. If one runs hard enough and long enough, one eventually catches the train. Once having caught the train, most people take a seat. A few will continue to move forward. As they edge closer to the front and peer off into the distance, they can begin to discern what is ahead, and where they may be going.

In order to facilitate such a chase, and to help others who have already boarded the train, we have assembled a group of highly qualified experts to cover particularly relevant topics including primary study design, statistical analysis, meta-analysis, consent and review board approval and the publication of research results. It is our expectation that the material covered should be of interest to both novice and experienced researchers. For those who choose to pursue a career that includes research, we can assure you that it is a great ride.

Finally, it may also be prudent to warn the unwary that being out in front can be perilous. If one stretches too far in front, one can fall (or be pushed) before the train!

Editors
Mark E. Brecher, MD
Michael P. Busch, MD, PhD

In: Brecher ME, Busch MP, eds.
Research Design and Analysis
Bethesda, MD: American Association of Blood Banks, 1998

1

Primary Study Design

James J. Korelitz, PhD, and
D. Robert Harris, PhD

IN ITS BROADEST INTERPRETATION, a study design can be defined as any systematic collection and interpretation of information. By this definition, a description of a case series or a collection of anecdotal reports could be considered a type of study design. In fact, the case series and anecdotal reports were the most commonly employed "study designs" in clinical research from the time of Hippocrates until as recently as the second half of the 20th century. While individual case descriptions can still be informative, the study designs used today tend to represent a more formal, systematic approach to: 1) defining the research questions and objectives prior to data collection; 2) collecting relevant, standardized information on exposure and outcome measures from a predefined, enumerated study population; 3) conducting appropriate statistical analyses; and 4) interpreting and reporting study results.

This chapter describes general categories and specific types of study designs, their advantages and disadvantages, and their use in three common research areas pertinent to blood banking and transfusion medicine. Also described are some practical issues associated with planning and conducting all types of study designs.

James J. Korelitz, PhD, Senior Epidemiologist and D. Robert Harris, PhD, Senior Study Director, Westat, Rockville, Maryland

General Categories of Study Designs

Different study designs can be categorized in a number of ways. Two qualities that help to describe the nature of a study are 1) whether it is a descriptive or analytic study, and 2) whether it is an experimental or observational study.

Descriptive vs Analytic Studies

As the name implies, the primary goal of a descriptive study is to describe a given population of subjects. For example, a study to estimate the prevalence of antibodies to human immunodeficiency virus type 1 (anti-HIV-1) among blood donors prior to screening[1] or a study to estimate the risk of transmission of HIV after screening tests were implemented[2] are descriptive studies. Certainly analytic techniques are required, but the main intent of the study is to describe the characteristics or status of the measured study group with the hope that the results apply to the larger population of interest. For example, estimates of transfusion-transmitted viral infections in one study population have been used to project the yield of nucleic acid amplification tests conducted on all blood donors in the United States.[3]

By contrast, an analytic study attempts to compare groups or assess associations between an exposure (beneficial or harmful) or risk factor and an outcome (positive or adverse). The focus of many analytic studies is specifically on whether a cause-and-effect relationship exists between an exposure or risk factor and the outcome of interest. The investigation of whether blood transfusions have the beneficial effect of reducing strokes in children with sickle cell disease[4] or whether blood transfusions have the adverse effect of inducing virus replication in HIV-1-infected people[5] are examples of analytic study designs.

The distinction between descriptive and analytic studies may not always be clear. A study whose objective is to estimate the prevalence of hepatitis C virus (HCV) among blood donors in a community might be called descriptive. Once the HCV prevalence is estimated, however, comparisons with the HCV prevalence in other communities (or in the same community at a different time) might be considered analytic. Labeling a study as descriptive or analytic is not as important as defining the study objectives clearly.

Experimental vs Observational Studies

The key distinguishing feature between experimental and observational studies is related to the assignment of exposure. Throughout this chapter, "exposure" is meant in the general sense of any potentially beneficial or harmful substance, clinical characteristic, or study factor that occurs prior to the outcome of interest. In an experimental study, the exposure is assigned to study subjects by the investigator. In an observational study, the exposure is not under the control of the investigator. Most experimental studies are analytic studies; that is, they are designed to compare the outcomes in groups of subjects who received different exposures. Observational studies are just as likely to be descriptive or analytic.

Many types of clinical trials are examples of experimental studies where the exposure represents a particular therapy or treatment. Subjects are assigned to various therapies by the investigator with the objective of comparing the efficacy of the different therapies. Many epidemiologic studies are examples of observational studies because the investigator does not assign exposure to subjects. In studies with human subjects, evaluations of the potentially harmful effects of an exposure or risk factor are usually observational due to ethical considerations that would preclude the investigator from exposing subjects to harmful substances. In observational studies, the subjects may have some influence on their exposure (eg, choice of occupation, intravenous drug use) or it may be totally out of the control of the subject (eg, genotype).

Specific Types of Study Designs

Most study designs can be classified into one of three types, depending on the order in which exposure and outcome data are obtained and examined—prospective, retrospective, and cross-sectional.

Prospective Studies

Perhaps the most straightforward and intuitive study design is the prospective (forward in time) study. These studies are also called cohort, longitudinal, or follow-up studies. Subjects are selected and classified according to their exposure status (eg, those with a risk factor and those without) or, in the case of an experimental study, an exposure is assigned (eg, some subjects receive treatment "A," and others receive treatment "B"). The two groups of subjects are then followed prospectively and the predefined outcome of interest is subsequently measured or observed (eg, cholesterol level, death). Comparisons are made between the exposure groups with the presumption that any observed difference in the outcome was caused by differences in the exposure.

The main advantages of a prospective study are the assurance that the exposure occurred prior to the outcome, and that subject selection is based solely on exposure without regard for or knowledge of the medical outcome of interest. Consequently, prospective studies are less prone to the outcome of interest affecting the availability or selection of subjects into the study. Also, prospective study designs may be necessary if the exposure is rare. In this case, subjects would be prescreened or identified by exposure status to ensure that an adequate number of exposed subjects were included in the study. The disadvantages of prospective studies include that: 1) it may take many years of follow-up time to observe the outcome of interest, 2) loss of subjects during this follow-up period can cause bias in the results, and 3) the cost can be greater than for other study designs due to the potentially larger number of subjects who need to be followed over an extended time, especially if the outcome is relatively uncommon.

Retrospective Studies

The criteria for selecting subjects and the order in which exposure and outcome data are collected for retrospective studies are the opposite of those for prospective studies. In a retrospective study, a group of subjects (cases) who already have the outcome of interest (eg, disease) is identified. For comparison, a group of subjects (controls) who are known not to have the outcome (eg, not diseased) is also selected. After the cases and controls have been selected, each group is examined or interviewed to determine its exposure status. If the exposure is more common in the diseased group than in the control group, then the implication is that an association between exposure and outcome exists. In a prospective study, the direction is forward. We ask, "Among those who are exposed, what proportion will subsequently develop the outcome?" In a retrospective study, the direction is backward. We ask, "Among those who already have the outcome, what proportion were previously exposed?" These retrospective studies are frequently called "case-control" or "case-referent" studies.

Case-control studies may be the only practical means for studying a rare outcome. They also offer the advantage of being able to provide a timely response to a research question because selecting subjects on the basis of their outcomes ensures that any latent period between the exposure and outcome has elapsed by the time the case-control study begins. The number of subjects required for valid statistical comparisons is usually less than the required sample size in prospective studies, which frequently translates into a lower cost for case-control studies. Potential methodologic problems associated with subject selection (eg, choosing an appropriate control group) and exposure assessment (eg, determining that exposure really occurred before the outcome, assessing whether subjects with the disease recall exposures differently than subjects without the disease) are the main drawbacks of the case-control design. Texts devoted to the design and analysis of case-control studies[6,7] should be consulted for further discussion of these important and complex matters.

Cross-Sectional Studies

In cross-sectional studies, sometimes called surveys or prevalence studies, subjects are selected for inclusion in the study without regard for either their exposure status (the defining feature of a prospective study) or outcome status (the defining attribute of a retrospective study). Instead, exposure or outcome information is obtained after subjects are determined to be eligible for the study. This information reflects the exposure and/or outcome status of the study population as it exists at a specific moment, or cross-section, of time.

If a representative sample is chosen, the cross-sectional study could be the most appropriate design for estimating the prevalence of one or more exposures or outcomes. It is especially useful in descriptive studies and for generating new hypotheses about an exposure-outcome relationship that could be examined later with a (generally more costly) prospective or retrospective study design. The main disadvantages of cross-sectional studies are their inability to reliably determine the temporal sequence of the exposure and outcome (similar to the limitation with case-control studies) and the possibility of subject selection bias that is inherent in relying on prevalent cases (eg, underrepresenting conditions with short durations or high mortality).

Study Designs Applied to Issues in Blood Banking and Transfusion Medicine

Three common research areas are of interest in blood banking and transfusion medicine. The areas are: 1) evaluating a new therapy or medical procedure, 2) evaluating a diagnostic or screening test, and 3) monitoring disease or disease markers. These areas are commonly thought of in the context of clinical and epidemiologic research, but the general philosophy and approach may also be of relevance in molecular studies.

Evaluating a Therapy or Procedure

The evaluation of a new therapy or medical procedure (hereafter referred to generically as a "treatment") usually begins with preclinical research, including animal testing, and proceeds to studies with human subjects in what has been called Phase I, II, III and IV studies in the drug development and regulatory fields.[8] Discussion of Phase I and II studies is beyond the scope of this chapter. Phase III studies are often the pivotal clinical trials that determine whether a treatment is approved, while Phase IV studies are sometimes called postmarketing studies that occur after a treatment is in widespread use. The key design considerations, however, are not related to whether the study is designated as Phase III or Phase IV. Rather, the principal design feature is the method by which a subject becomes part of the treatment group or comparison group. Thus, the primary distinction is whether the study is experimental or observational in nature.

Clinical Trials (Experimental)

Most clinical trials are analytic, experimental, and prospective in nature. They are analytic because the primary objective is to compare outcomes between groups that received different treatments (ie, to evaluate whether a cause-and-effect relationship exists between a treatment and an outcome). They are experimental because the investigator assigns the treatment to each participating patient, and they are prospective because the subjects are then followed prospectively over time to determine their outcomes. A study to compare different types of platelet transfusions on subsequent formation of antiplatelet alloantibodies and refractoriness to platelet transfusions[9] and a study to compare different methods for reducing the risk of transfusion-associated cytomegalovirus[10] are examples of clinical trials. In both cases, the type of treatment (ie, the transfused product) was assigned to each subject by the study investigator.

A study where the investigator selects a treatment for a subject based on clinical judgment, however, is not much different than one where subjects determine their own exposure or treatment, ie, an observational study. A critical component of a properly designed experimental study is the *random* assignment of treatments to the study groups. Although a subject may be required to meet certain well-defined inclusion criteria in order to be considered eligible for the study (eg, to be within a specific age range, to have a certain diagnostic classification or stage of disease, etc), once it is established that these criteria are met the assignment to different treatment groups should be based on a random process. Random assignment to treatment groups ensures that allocation bias is avoided. Investigators should not be allowed to consciously or subconsciously assign a subject to a preferred treatment group, as there might be a tendency to assign a certain type of patient (ie, with either more severe or less severe disease) to the treatment being investigated and thereby influence the outcome of the study. Random assignment also makes it likely (although it does not guarantee) that the treatment groups will be comparable on other factors (ie, confounding factors) that may affect the outcome, including factors that may not have been previously known to be associated with the outcome.

Furthermore, random assignment is the basis for subsequently being able to make formal probability statements about the likelihood that a treatment effect exists. The different manners and actual logistics for making random assignments (eg, adaptive, stratified, block, etc) can be found in standard texts on clinical trials.[11,12] Study designs that compare subjects from multiple facilities where different treatment methods are used as the standard of care are not formal experimental designs. Likewise, designs that randomly assign use of a particular treatment to clinical sites for all of their patients do not qualify as truly experimental, as there may be inherent institutional differences that confound the evaluation of the treatment effect.[13] Random assignment to a treatment group should be made at the individual patient level.

The above discussion on random assignment implies the existence of a comparison group. The comparison group usually receives an inactive compound (ie, a placebo) or is treated with the prevailing standard of care. It also implies that subjects were randomly assigned to either the treatment group or a comparison group and were then followed during approximately the same calendar period. This type of concurrent control group is generally preferred. Sometimes, historical controls are used as a comparison group. The experience of subjects from previous studies or from medical records is used to form the control group. This method has the practical advantages of being quicker and less expensive to complete, and the potential ethical advantage of assigning the new treatment to all new study subjects. While historical controls are listed in the Food and Drug Administration (FDA) regulations (21 CFR 314.126) as a potential source for a control group, they should be used only for special circumstances. The possible biases from historical controls could be severe if the characteristics of the patients or the standard of care have changed since the time data were collected on the historical control group.

Not only should the treatment be assigned randomly, but also whenever possible, it should be administered blindly.[12] A single-blind study means that the study subjects do not know to which treatment group they have been assigned. This is particularly important if the outcomes of interest are patient-reported events, such as symptoms. In a double-blind study, neither the subject nor the investigator is aware of whether the subject is part of the treatment or the control group. The randomized, placebo-controlled, double-blind, clinical trial is generally considered the ideal experimental design. Explanations of more complicated types of clinical trial designs, such as cross-over, Latin square, and factorial designs can be found elsewhere.[14]

The goal of a clinical trial is to determine whether a treatment "works," which is evaluated by answering two questions: 1) Is it safe? and 2) Is it efficacious? Frequently, the objective is to measure whether a new treatment has greater efficacy than an existing treatment, while being equally safe. Sometimes the hypothesis of the study states that the new treatment is equally as efficacious as the standard of care but is safer to use (ie, has fewer adverse side effects). Or, a study could be designed to test whether a new treatment that is easier or less costly to administer is equally as safe and efficacious as the existing standard. The design considerations are basically the same regardless of the specific research objective. But, there may be different statistical issues, including sample size and power estimates, depending on whether a study is trying to measure a benefit or assess equivalency. In any case, in the United States, a new treatment is not approved by the FDA unless there is convincing evidence (often from at least two randomized placebo-controlled double-blind studies) that it is safe and efficacious. Comprehensive discussions covering many of the issues faced in designing and conducting clinical trials can be found in several texts.[8,12,15-17]

Epidemiologic Studies (Observational)

If randomized placebo-controlled double-blind Phase III clinical trials have already established the safety and efficacy of a treatment, one might question whether any additional studies are necessary. The answer is derived by examining more closely the characteristics of randomized controlled trials. Regarding safety, a Phase III trial may have included no more than several hundred subjects. Rare adverse events that occur with a frequency of only 1 in 1000 or 1 in 10,000 people are unlikely to be detected in a Phase III clinical trial. Yet, even this low incidence might be considered unacceptably high if the adverse event is severe (eg, permanent disability or death). Second, a Phase III trial typically is of short duration, frequently lasting less than 1-2 years, and sometimes only a matter of weeks. Therefore, it is impossible to assess the consequences of long-term use of a treatment, or even the long-term effects of short-term use. Third, the eligibility requirements for subjects to enroll in a Phase III trial are often quite restrictive. Frequently, a homogeneous study group is desired to allow the treatment effect to be assessed more directly. The result, however, is that subgroups that may be adversely affected by the treatment may not be identified because they were not included in the study.

Regarding efficacy, a Phase III trial is conducted under very controlled conditions. In practice, people may not be as compliant with the recommended treatment regimen or may not be followed as closely by their physician. The true *effectiveness* of a treatment in "real world" applications may be different than the *efficacy* measured in a controlled clinical trial. As a consequence, additional broad-based population studies of a treatment may be warranted with a more diverse study population to confirm the findings observed from earlier clinical trials.

The terms "Phase IV study," "postmarketing surveillance," and "pharmacoepidemiology" are frequently associated with clinical epidemiologic studies. Whereas clinical trials tend to be categorized similarly (ie, analytic, experimental, and prospective), epidemiologic studies can be descriptive or analytic, and prospective, retrospective, or cross-sectional. They also can be observational or experimental. It is much more common, however, for epidemiologic studies to be observational (ie, the investigator does not have the opportunity to randomly assign subjects into exposure or treatment groups). Because epidemiologic studies are so frequently observational studies, the two terms are often considered synonymous.

Epidemiologic studies generally attempt to describe health-related outcomes with respect to person, place, and time. These studies examine the classical who, what, when, and where questions. Who is affected (which people or subgroups experience higher or lower outcome rates, or what personal characteristics increase or decrease the likelihood of being affected)? What is occurring (describing the natural history or clinical course)? When is it occurring (timing, secular changes)? Where is it occurring (geographic patterns, clusters)? Epidemiologic studies tend to involve large, diverse groups of people. Fundamentals of epidemiologic concepts and methods can be found in several texts.[18,19]

Prospective epidemiologic studies bear the closest resemblance to clinical trials. Again, the key distinction is that the investigator does not randomly assign the treatment or exposure to subjects in observational studies. For example, the Transfusion-Transmitted Viruses Study (TTVS)[20] was a prospective study of transfusion-associated diseases. The study included prospective follow-up of hospital patients who received blood transfusion (ie, the "exposed" group) and a control group of hospital patients who did not receive blood transfusion (ie, the "unexposed" group). This study is considered observational, or noninterventional, because whether transfusions were administered depended on clinical need, and not on a randomization procedure. The comparison of long-term mortality rates in transfusion recipients who did and did not have transfusion-associated hepatitis[21] and the comparison of postoperative mortality among subjects who did and did not receive perioperative blood transfusions[22] are also examples of prospective, observational studies. Although the study cohorts for these two studies were assembled from past medical records, both studies are considered prospective designs because subjects were selected based on exposure (ie, whether they had posttransfusion hepatitis and whether they received perioperative blood transfusions) and followed prospectively to determine their outcome (ie, mortality).

Retrospective epidemiologic studies are also seen in blood banking and transfusion medicine research. The examination of potential risk factors for human T-cell lymphotropic virus types I and II (HTLV-I and -II) in blood donors was a retrospective (case-control) study.[23] People who were anti-HTLV positive were identified through screening of blood donors, and a group of controls who were known to be seronegative for anti-HTLV was selected. Persons in each group were then interviewed about their past potential HTLV risk factors. A study that showed no association between Creutzfeldt-Jakob disease (CJD) and previous surgery or blood transfusion, or consumption of beef, veal, lamb, cheese, or milk[24] used a retrospective study design. This was determined by selecting subjects (cases) because they had been diagnosed with CJD and comparing their past exposures to subjects (controls) who were selected because they did not have CJD.

Cross-sectional epidemiologic studies also are commonly used in this field. For example, a telephone survey of blood donor attitudes on donation-related issues[25] and the assessment of HCV prevalence and genotype distribution in volunteer blood donors[26] are examples of cross-sectional study designs. In each case, the study group was selected and measured at a single cross-section of time.

Evaluating a Diagnostic or Screening Test

The purpose of a diagnostic or screening test is to correctly classify people into two categories: those with the health-related outcome or condition of interest (hereafter referred to generically as "disease") and those without the disease. The classification is usually based on the numerical results of the diagnostic test relative to a chosen cutoff point; results greater than the cutoff point are considered "positive" and results at or below the cutoff point are labeled "negative" (or vice versa). The presumption is that people with a positive diagnostic test result have the disease and people with negative test results do not have the disease. The degree to which this is true is the basis for evaluating the validity of the diagnostic or screening test.

The validity of a diagnostic test is quantified by estimating its sensitivity and specificity. Sensitivity is defined as the percentage of diseased people who have positive test results. Specificity is defined as the percentage of nondiseased people who have negative test results. These two parameters are formally determined by specially designed clinical trials. For these trials, a group of subjects (or specimens) who are known to have the disease is selected. The percentage of positive test results measured within this group provides an estimate of the test's sensitivity. A group of subjects who are known not to have the disease is also selected. The percentage of negative test results measured within this group provides an estimate of the test's specificity.

Other features of a diagnostic or screening test that need to be addressed also can be thought of in terms of sensitivity and specificity. For example, determining the detection limit of an assay is a matter of sensitivity (in fact, it is sometimes called the assay's analytic sensitivity) among a select group of subjects who are known to be infected. The question can be phrased as, "Among subjects who are known to contain a specific amount of detectable material (eg, viral or bacterial particles), what percent will test positive?" Or, equivalently, "What amount of detectable material must be present in a subject in order for there to be a sufficiently high probability that it will test positive?" Likewise, determining the number of days after an infection that a person will produce a positive test result (or the number of days earlier than an existing screening test) is a matter of sensitivity calculated within a special subgroup of recently infected subjects. Whether there are certain interfering substances that tend to produce false-negative test results is also a matter of sensitivity within a specific type of specimen. Conditions associated with false-positive test results are relevant to fully characterizing a test's specificity. Even issues of stability and reproducibility reduce to the same questions. Will a diseased person consistently test positive (if the specimen is collected, stored, and handled in a particular way)? Will a nondiseased person consistently test negative? Therefore, the evaluation of the performance of a diagnostic test is not a matter of calculating a single set of values for the test's sensitivity and specificity. It also requires an examination of the types of specimens and conditions that are associated with an increased chance of a false-positive test result (ie, decreased specificity) or false-negative test result (ie, decreased sensitivity).

Note that the study design described above is an example of a retrospective study—a group of subjects who already have the outcome of interest (eg, a disease) is identified, and for comparison a group of subjects who are known not to have the outcome is also selected. The exposure, in this case, is a positive diagnostic test result. The classical retrospective study asks, "Among those who already have the outcome, what percentage were exposed?" This is equivalent to asking, "What is the sensitivity of a diagnostic test?"

As stated in the description of a retrospective study, the direction of the question, "Among those with the disease, what percentage will have positive test results?" is backwards. Of greater relevance is the (forward) question, "Among those who have positive test results, what percentage have the disease?" The answer to that question is known as the positive predictive value of the test. At first glance, it may appear that only a trivial recalculation of available data needs to be made in order to answer this question. For example, consider the results of a clinical trial shown in Table 1-1. The study consisted of 1000 subjects who were known to have the disease. Among this group, 900 tested positive (ie, the test's sensitivity was 90%). The study also included 1000 subjects who were known not to have the disease. Among this group, 950 tested negative (ie, the test's specificity was 95%). The answer to the question, "Among those who had positive test results, what percentage had the disease?" seems simply to be

Table 1-1. Example of Sensitivity, Specificity, and Positive Predictive Value of a Screening Test, Disease Prevalence = 50% (1000/2000)

Screening Test	Disease Yes	Disease No	Total
Positive	900	50	950
Negative	100	950	1050
Total	1000	1000	2000

Sensitivity = 900/(900 + 100) = 90%
Specificity = 950/(50 + 950) = 95%
Positive Predictive Value = 900/(900 + 50) = 94.7 %

900/(900+50) = 94.7%. For the clinical trial to represent what will actually be observed in practice, however, it is necessary that the study population accurately reflects the prevalence of disease that will be encountered in the general community. The example in Table 1-1 states that the disease prevalence is 50% (1000/2000). In order to obtain an accurate assessment of sensitivity, clinical trials of diagnostic tests typically include a much greater percentage of people with the disease than would be found in the general population. As shown in Table 1-2, if the same diagnostic test (with 90% sensitivity and 95% specificity) is used in a population where the prevalence of disease is 5%, then the positive predictive value will drop to 48.7%. In the blood donor setting, the prevalence of infectious disease markers can be significantly less than 5%. For example, the prevalence of HCV is approximately 3 per 1000 (0.3%).[27] A test with 95% sensitivity and 99.9% specificity will have a positive predictive value of 74%; that is, 26% of people with *positive* HCV test results will *not* be infected.

Although a test might be thought of as yielding only a positive or negative test result, it will usually have a numerical component (eg, optical density, absorbance value, relative light units) and a decision must be made to select a cutoff point value for making the dichotomous designation. In some

Table 1-2. Example of Sensitivity, Specificity, and Positive Predictive Value of a Screening Test, Disease Prevalence = 5% (100/2000)

Screening Test	Disease Yes	Disease No	Total
Positive	90	95	185
Negative	10	1805	1815
Total	100	1900	2000

Sensitivity = 90/(90 + 10) = 90%
Specificity = 1805/(95 + 1805) = 95%
Positive Predictive Value = 90/(90+95) = 48.7%

situations, the test results in people with the disease will be completely different than those in people without the disease. Assays for infectious diseases typically produce numerical values that cluster at opposite ends of a scale, and selecting a distinguishing cutoff point value is not difficult (there may still be false-positive and false-negative results, but they are not dependent on the choice of the cutoff point value). In other situations, however, people with and without the disease may have overlapping distributions of test results. For example, high alanine aminotransferase (ALT) levels are associated with liver disease, but there is not one obvious ALT cutoff point that clearly separates those with and without liver disease. Under these conditions, the choice of a cutoff point for classifying people as positive (ie, diseased) or negative (ie, not diseased) forces a decision to be made regarding the trade-off between sensitivity and specificity. Setting the cutoff point higher will reduce sensitivity but increase specificity. Lowering the cutoff point will increase sensitivity but decrease specificity. The effect that different cutoff points have on the observed sensitivity and specificity can be summarized by generating the receiver-operating characteristic (ROC) curve, where sensitivity is plotted against one-minus-specificity over a range of possible cutoff point values.[28]

The calculation of sensitivity and specificity, as previously described, depends on knowing the true status of each study subject and comparing the diagnostic test result with the true status. While the actual calculations of sensitivity and specificity are simple, the true status of a subject may be difficult to assess, as it implies that a criterion standard, or "gold standard," exists for making that determination. Sometimes, a criterion standard is not available due to practical or ethical reasons (eg, more definitive testing is too costly to be performed on all subjects, or an invasive technique is required to confirm disease status). In these circumstances, the new diagnostic test may be compared to the results from the existing standard. Because the existing standard may not be perfect, it is sometimes referred to as an "alloyed standard." Follow-up testing may then be used to resolve the subset of results where discrepancies were observed between the new diagnostic test and the alloyed standard. Under certain conditions, this type of discrepant (or discordant) analysis can lead to biased estimates of a test's performance.[29,30]

Finally, the reason for performing a diagnostic or screening test must be considered as part of its evaluation. The purpose of a test may be to "screen out" infectious blood, tissue, or organs. Or, the purpose may be to "screen in" asymptomatic patients who may have, or be at increased risk of acquiring, a medical condition and who would benefit from early diagnosis and treatment. Also, a screening test might be used as the basis for quantifying and monitoring the prevalence or incidence of a disease within a community (as opposed to a clinical diagnosis within an individual) as part of a surveillance program. In each of these examples, the basic methods for evaluating the test's performance are the same. However, the consequences of false-positive and false-negative test results may be different. For example, the acceptance of a test system that uses saliva specimens as an alternative to serum specimens for anti-HIV testing might depend on whether it is intended as a blood donor screening test or a public health surveillance tool.[31] Hence, determining acceptable levels and relative importance of a test's sensitivity vs its specificity will depend on the setting in which the screening test is applied.

Monitoring Disease (Surveillance)

A third area of research in blood banking and transfusion medicine research relates to monitoring the occurrence or frequency of an event or characteristic of interest. Most commonly, this refers to the surveillance of health outcomes (eg, diseases, adverse events), but risk factors for diseases also can be monitored, either by a single cross-sectional survey[32] or through an ongoing surveillance system.[33,34] The emphasis of the remainder of this section is on disease surveillance.

The primary aim of disease surveillance is to quantify how often a disease occurs. In addition to being able to assess the potential current public health impact of a particular disease, a surveillance program might address such important questions as: What is the pattern in the number of cases reported over time (eg, are there long-term secular trends, is there an acute outbreak)? Are there particular geographic areas where the disease is occurring more frequently (or less frequently) than in other places? Are there more cases being reported in certain demographic subgroups of people? Obtaining such information for transfusion-associated infectious disease markers in a community is of obvious relevance to the blood banking professional.

The type of study design used for disease or disease marker surveillance depends on the specific research objectives, but is most commonly cross-sectional in nature. A surveillance system might not seem compatible with a cross-sectional design. Surveillance implies an ongoing monitoring of disease, suggesting that a prospective study design might be appropriate. In contrast, data collected from cross-sectional study designs are associated with a single point in time. Although a prospective design might be preferred, a cross-sectional design is more practical. A prospective surveillance system would require that a specific group of subjects be identified and followed over time. This can be approximated with a series of multiple cross-sectional studies. Furthermore, the goal of the surveillance system may be to monitor disease occurrence within a particular geographic area. If so, periodic cross-sectional studies in the same geographic area will be a better reflection of potential changes in disease prevalence in that area than continuing to follow a cohort, some members of which might migrate out of the area.

Many surveillance systems do not use a well-defined, explicitly enumerated study cohort. Instead, there is only the implication that the study group exists. Often, the study cohort is assumed to be all people living within the same geographic boundary or catchment area that gave rise to the reported cases, but the actual identification of all eligible study subjects is not made. This is a marked contrast from the study designs previously discussed, and is closer in design to a series of case reports. For some surveillance purposes, the lack of a formal, prespecified study group does not pose a problem. For example, a surveillance system may be able to accurately estimate the prevalence of a disease even if it only collects information on the number of cases that are reported within a certain geographic area. In order to obtain the needed denominator for the prevalence calculation, an external data source (eg, census information) may be available. In this case, the prevalence of a disease also could be estimated among demographic subgroups, assuming both the case reports and census information contain demographic data. If a denominator is not available, the numerator (ie, number of reported cases) alone could provide a useful indicator of disease occurrence. If it is assumed that the denominator is constant, then even if its value is not known, an increase in the number of cases would imply that the incidence of disease is increasing. This assumption is more likely to hold for short periods, making it possible to identify acute outbreaks (but making secular trends difficult to confirm). Information collected only on cases reported to a surveillance system may be sufficient to characterize the clinical features of affected individuals and describe the natural history of a disease.[35] Also, these cases could be used to form the basis for subsequent case-control studies.[36]

The lack of a predefined, enumerated study group, however, can create certain limitations to surveillance systems. While some surveillance systems are based on active reporting systems that include methods for assessing whether all eligible cases are identified, others rely solely on passive, volunteer reporting procedures.[37] Even with active reporting systems, the investigator generally has less control over the evaluation and diagnosis of reported cases. As a consequence, surveillance systems can be subject to reporting artifacts caused by changes in referral and reporting patterns. Surveillance systems based on prevailing medical practice, rather than on fixed, standardized procedures specified in a study protocol, also will be affected by changes in diagnostic tests. For example, the apparent increase in the occurrence of HCV in blood donors between 1991 and 1993 was a reflection of the change from the first-generation to second-generation anti-HCV screening test, and not due to an acute outbreak of HCV in blood donors.[38,39] Also, critical supplemental patient information that normally would be collected on case report forms in a clinical trial may not be routinely available from reports collected by a surveillance system. For example, a surveillance system based on spontaneous adverse event reports might not contain complete information on a patient's relevant clinical history, thus limiting the ability to make statements about a potential cause-and-effect relationship between a drug and an adverse event.

Therefore, many surveillance systems serve as a means for generating an initial signal that a potential problem may exist. The FDA's Medical Products Reporting Program (MedWatch) and Adverse Event Reporting System (AERS) are examples of surveillance systems designed to capture information generated from spontaneous reports submitted by health-care providers. The results tend to be more descriptive in nature than analytic and are more likely to generate hypotheses than to test them. The information from a surveillance system can help to direct resources to appropriate areas (both in terms of geography and subject matter) and to plan formal analytic studies.

Planning and Conducting Studies

Many of the tasks associated with planning and conducting a study are common to all study designs. For example, ensuring that sufficient funds are available to conduct the study is a universal requirement. The following sections are a sample of other aspects of planning and conducting a study that are relevant, regardless of study design.

Writing a Protocol

The study protocol represents the blueprint for conducting the study. From descriptive, observational studies to randomized, placebo-controlled, double-blind, clinical trials, the study protocol documents the general design as well as many of the details of the study. An opening section on background and general purpose leads into the specific study objectives (and hypotheses to be tested if it is an analytic study). The study population must be identified and subject inclusion/exclusion criteria defined. The number of subjects that will be required in order to obtain estimates and comparisons with a predefined level of precision should be determined from statistical power calculations and presented in the protocol. If a treatment or intervention is planned, the protocol will describe the assignment (preferably random) of subjects to a treatment/intervention, along with the details of its administration. If the study is observational, the methods for assessing exposure (which may be a therapy selected by a subject or physician) are specified. For all study designs, the outcome measure(s) (including possible follow-up evaluations of study subjects) need to be clearly defined in the protocol. The logistics of collecting data are specified in the protocol, usually through the inclusion of copies of the data forms (eg, case report forms) that will be used and an explanation of how to complete and process the forms (a separate manual of procedures may be necessary if the study is complex). The protocol should state study monitoring and other quality assurance measures used throughout the study to make sure that the procedures given in the protocol are followed. The protocol should address informed consent plans and other ethical issues that may be relevant, as well as administrative issues such as the organizational structure and responsibilities of investigators participating in the study. Finally, a statistical plan is included to describe how the data will be analyzed. With some clinical trials, the exact means for conducting interim analyses while the study is in progress and for using those results to decide whether to continue the trial must be stated. The following four sections further discuss selected issues that should be addressed in the protocol.

Selecting a Study Population

The study population is defined in the protocol and represents the subjects (or specimens) who are eligible for inclusion in the study. The study population is distinct from the target population and the study sample. The target population is the broader group to which the investigator will extrapolate the study results. The study sample is the subset of the study population that contributes the data that are analyzed in the study. The subjects in the study sample may differ from the study population if subjects who are otherwise eligible refuse to participate in the study, are lost to follow-up, or for some other reason have unusable data. Ideally, the participation and compliance rates will be very high so that the number of subjects and the characteristics of the study sample will be very close to the study population.

Defining the appropriate study population so that it reflects the experience of the target population is a more problematic issue. With clinical trials in particular, the study population is often intentionally restricted to a very narrow and homogeneous group of people defined by a long list of inclusion and exclusion criteria. The advantage of this strategy is that the treatment effect can be estimated without potential extraneous factors affecting the assessment. For example, the protocol for a clinical trial of a therapeutic agent for the treatment of a particular disease may require that subjects not have other diseases and/or that they not be taking concomitant medications. The target population, however, may be all people with the disease under study, regardless of other diseases they may have or other medications they may be taking. In this case, the study population may not be representative of the target population. The evaluation of a diagnostic, or screening test is susceptible to this problem. The sensitivity of the test to detect an infection or a disease should be conducted on subjects from the full clinical and pathological spectrum of patients on whom the test is intended to be used. The control group, used to evaluate the test's specificity, also should be similar to people who will be tested. For a diagnostic test, this might mean selecting people with similar clinical symptoms (but who do not have the disease of interest) rather than completely asymptomatic people.

Collecting Information

Another feature common to all study designs is the systematic collection of information that will be used to address the research questions. In some studies, data collection may be under the control of the investigators to the extent that they may be able to dictate which data items are to be measured. In other studies, the investigators may be restricted to accessing and abstracting information that has already been obtained and recorded in medical charts or other information sources. In both instances, data collection forms should be designed to efficiently capture the data items required for the study. These forms should facilitate the data processing and quality assurance procedures that are needed to produce the data files that will be used for subsequent statistical analyses.

A distinction is sometimes made between the quality of so-called "hard" or objective data and "soft" or subjective data. Objective data are derived from an object, such as an instrument or equipment. They are commonly thought of in terms of numerical values (eg, grams per liter of hemoglobin, copies per milliliter of HIV-1 RNA), but they could also be categorical (eg, blood type) or dichotomous (positive/negative). Subjective data are obtained from the response of a subject or other observer. These data are frequently categorical or dichotomous responses to questions about symptoms, medical history, or personal characteristics (eg, yes/no answers to questions about shortness of breath or past intravenous drug use), but they could also be numerical (eg, number of missed work days).

With both objective and subjective data, however, the investigator needs to evaluate potential biases that may exist within the collected information. These biases may arise for a number of reasons. With "soft" data the problem of recall bias is relevant, especially in case-control studies or unblinded prospective studies. Subjects with a disease (the cases in case-control studies) may recall past exposures either more accurately (they are more motivated to remember) or less accurately (they may have preconceived ideas about what caused their illness) than the controls. Subjects taking a known therapy (the treated group in an unblinded prospective study) may report fewer symptoms than the control group for artificial reasons (eg, they are hesitant to complain about a promising new drug). Subjects may intentionally, or unintentionally, report inaccurate information to an interviewer or record it on a self-administered questionnaire for a variety of reasons (eg, desire to please, misunderstanding the question, fear of releasing personally sensitive information).

Objective data are sometimes considered more valid than subjective data because quantitative results are obtained from a machine readout. Nevertheless, underlying the numerical value (sometimes reported with great precision) there can be many sources of uncertainty or variability. Different operators of test equipment following the same testing procedures can produce different results on the same specimen. Likewise, the same technologist can get different results on the same subject or specimen tested at different times. Variations in reagents used for an assay or differences in the collection, storage, and handling of specimens can cause widely different results. Also, there might be significant biological variability within a subject depending on the time of day a measurement or specimen was taken or other characteristics (eg, fasting vs nonfasting, overall state of health). Thus, data that appear on the surface to be "hard" should not automatically be assumed to be more reliable than "soft" data. Furthermore, if quality-of-life issues are important in the assessment of health, subjective outcomes such as the relief of symptoms may be more relevant than a particular quantitative test result such as a 10% increase in platelet count.

Analysis and Reporting of Results

The analysis of data collected during a study and reporting of the results are required of all study designs. The primary endpoints to be evaluated and the statistical plan for conducting the analyses should be defined in the study protocol before data collection begins. In addition to the main effect under investigation, potential sources of bias from extraneous, or confounding, variables should be taken into account by the analysis plan (eg, through stratification, multivariable models). Often, more than one analytic approach may be valid for a study. Multiple analytic approaches that produce similar conclusions can provide some assurance that the findings are not a statistical artifact of a particular methodology. When formal statistical comparisons are made, it is preferable to provide a confidence interval for a given estimate rather than stating only whether a statistical test is significant (eg, $p<0.05$). The confidence interval reflects both the magnitude and precision of the estimated effect. Explanations of the theory and techniques related to statistical analyses can be found in numerous textbooks,[40-42] as well as in Chapter 3 which includes a detailed discussion of statistical testing and the interpretation of p-values.

The requirement for analysis and reporting of results also pertains to studies that do not show a treatment effect or an association between a hypothesized risk factor and health outcome. These studies are sometimes given the unfortunate misnomer of "negative studies." However, any well-designed and properly conducted study makes a positive contribution to the scientific knowledge base regardless of the results. Although there may be a tendency on the part of researchers and journal editors to give more attention to studies that show statistically significant results, it is important to include the findings from all well-conducted studies when attempting to produce a weight-of-evidence assessment of a particular topic. This issue is further addressed in Chapter 2.

Ethical Issues

The use of human subjects in medical research experiments is an important and sensitive matter. When two (or more) therapies or procedures are already considered part of the acceptable standard of care, conducting a clinical trial to formally compare these different methods does not seem to pose an ethical problem. The use of human subjects in medical studies to evaluate whether a new therapy is safe and effective, however, raises an obvious question. Is it ethical to give an unproven therapy to a person? It may also be relevant to ask whether it is ethical to give a placebo to a person?[43,44]

Many of the issues concerning the use of human subjects are dealt with in policies stated by the US Department of Health and Human Services, National Institutes of Health, Office for Protection from Research Risks and published in the *Code of Federal Regulations* (45 CFR 46). While these regulations apply to studies conducted or supported by a federal department or agency, they are also relevant to non-government-funded studies. Two key components of a system to ensure ethical use of human subjects in research studies are: 1) a process for obtaining informed consent from each study participant (with special considerations for certain populations such as children, pregnant women, and prisoners), and 2) review of the study protocol by an outside, independent, review board. Each of these components is covered in Chapter 4.

Summary

Study designs used in research today are significantly more complex than the case-series reports of the past. Collections of individual case reports still serve an important role in raising suspicions about potential cause-and-effect relationships. More rigorous study designs are generally needed, however, to resolve issues related to the safety and effectiveness of a therapy or procedure, or to identify and quantify the hazard of a particular risk factor, exposure, or personal trait.

An important characteristic distinguishing study designs involves the investigator's role in assigning treatments/exposures to study subjects; studies that use a random assignment method are called experimental, and all others are called observational. The basis for selecting study subjects is another fundamental study design consideration; studies that first determine (or assign) exposure and subsequently measure the outcome are prospective designs, while studies that select subjects because they already have the outcome of interest (and a group of control subjects who do not) and subsequently obtain past exposure information are retrospective designs. Cross-sectional designs tend to measure exposures, outcomes, or both as they exist at a single point in time.

Within the general categories of experimental/observational and prospective/retrospective/cross-sectional studies are numerous variations and hybrid designs. For all studies, it is essential to develop a written protocol that states the research objectives and defines all the requirements of the study design (subject eligibility, definition of endpoint, etc). The protocol is used to help standardize the methods and procedures used throughout the study period, which is an especially critical need of multicenter studies. Furthermore, after the study has been completed, the protocol provides information (more than can be included in a journal article) about the study design and implementation details that are needed to compare the results to those from other studies and to plan future studies that will logically build upon the foundation laid by previous research.

References

1. Kleinman SH, Nilan JC, Azen SP, et al. Prevalence of antibodies to human immunodeficiency virus type 1 among blood donors prior to screening. Transfusion 1989;29: 572-80.
2. Lackritz EM, Satten GA, Aberle-Grasse J, et al. Estimated risk of transmission of the human immunodeficiency virus by screened blood in the United States. N Engl J Med 1995;333:1721-5.
3. Schreiber GB, Busch MP, Kleinman SH, Korelitz JJ. The risk of transfusion-transmitted viral infections. N Engl J Med 1996;334:1685-90.

4. Adams RJ, McKie VC, Brambilla D, et al. Stroke prevention trial in sickle cell anemia. Control Clin Trials 1998; 19:110-29.
5. Busch MP, Collier A, Gernsheimer T, et al. The Viral Activation Transfusion Study (VATS): Rationale, objectives, and design overview. Transfusion 1996;36:854-9.
6. Breslow NE, Day NE. Statistical methods in cancer research, vol 1. The analysis of case-control studies. Lyon: International Agency for Research on Cancer, 1980.
7. Schlesselman JJ. Case-control studies. New York: Oxford University Press, 1982.
8. Pocock SJ. Clinical trials: A practical approach. Chichester: Wiley, 1983.
9. The Trial to Reduce Alloimmunization to Platelets Study Group. Leukocyte reduction and ultraviolet B irradiation of platelets to prevent alloimmunization and refractoriness to platelet transfusions. N Engl J Med 1997;337: 1861-9.
10. Bowden RA, Slichter SJ, Sayers M, et al. A comparison of filtered leukocyte-reduced and cytomegalovirus (CMV) seronegative blood products for the prevention of transfusion-associated CMV infection after marrow transplant. Blood 1995;86:3598-603.
11. Friedman LM, Furberg CD, DeMets DL. Fundamentals of clinical trials, 3rd ed. St. Louis: Mosby-Year Book, 1996.
12. Meinert CL, Tonascia S. Clinical trials: Design, conduct, and analysis. New York: Oxford University Press, 1986.
13. Surgenor DM, Churchill WH, Wallace EL, et al. The specific hospital significantly affects red cell and component transfusion practice in coronary artery bypass graft surgery: A study of five hospitals. Transfusion 1998;38:122-34.
14. Fleiss JL. The design and analysis of clinical experiments. New York: Wiley, 1986.
15. Piantadosi S. Clinical trials: A methodologic perspective. New York: Wiley, 1997.
16. Thall PF. Recent advances in clinical trial design and analysis. Boston: Kluwer Academic Publishers, 1995.
17. Hulley SB, Cummings SR. Designing clinical research. Baltimore: Williams and Wilkins, 1988.
18. Rothman KJ, Greenland S. Modern epidemiology, 2nd ed. Philadelphia: Lippincott-Raven, 1998.

19. Kelsey JL, Whittemore AS, Evans AS, Thompson WD. Methods in observational epidemiology, 2nd ed. New York: Oxford University Press, 1996.
20. Holland PV, Bancroft W, Zimmerman H. Post-transfusion viral hepatitis and the TTVS. N Engl J Med 1981;304:1033-5.
21. Seeff LB, Buskell-Bales Z, Wright EC, et al. Long-term mortality after transfusion-associated non-A, non-B hepatitis. N Engl J Med 1992;327:1906-11.
22. Carson JL, Duff A, Berlin JA, et al. Perioperative blood transfusion and postoperative mortality. JAMA 1998; 279:199-205.
23. Schreiber GB, Murphy EL, Horton JA, et al. Risk factor for human T-cell lymphotropic virus types I and II in blood donors: The Retrovirus Epidemiology Donor Study. J Acquir Immune Defic Syndr 1997;14:263-71.
24. van Duijn CM, Delasniere-Lauprêtre N, Masullo C, et al. Case-control study of risk factors of Creutzfeldt-Jakob disease in Europe during 1993-95. Lancet 1998;351:1081-4.
25. Bowman RJ, Clay ME, Therkelsen DJ, et al. Donor attitudes about exporting and importing blood. Transfusion 1997;37:913-20.
26. Mison LM, Young IF, O'Donoghue M, et al. Prevalence of hepatitis C virus and genotype distributions in an Australian volunteer blood donor population. Transfusion 1997;37:73-8.
27. Murphy EL, Bryzman S, Williams AE, et al. Demographic determinants of hepatitis C virus seroprevalence among blood donors. JAMA 1996;275:995-1000.
28. Zweig MH, Campbell G. Receiver-operating characteristic (ROC) plots: A fundamental evaluation tool in clinical medicine. Clin Chem 1993;39:561-77.
29. Miller WC. Bias in discrepant analysis: When two wrongs don't make a right. J Clin Epidemiol 1998;51:219-31.
30. Hadgu A. The discrepancy in discrepant analysis. Lancet 1996;348:592-3.
31. Gallo D, George JR, Fitchen JH, et al. Evaluation of a system using oral mucosal transudate for HIV-1 antibody screening and confirmatory testing. JAMA 1997;277:254-8.

32. Williams AE, Thomson RA, Schreiber GB, et al. Estimates of infectious disease risk factors in US blood donors. JAMA 1997;277:967-72.
33. Remington PL, Smith MY, Williamson DF, et al. Design, characteristics, and usefulness of state-based behavioral risk factor surveillance: 1981-1987. Public Health Rep 1988;103:366-75.
34. Powell-Griner E, Anderson JE, Murphy W. State- and sex-specific prevalence of selected characteristics—behavior risk factor surveillance system, 1994-1995. MMWR CDC Surveill Summ 1997;46:1-31.
35. Alter MJ, Margolis HS, Krawczynski K, et al. The natural history of community-acquired hepatitis C in the United States. N Engl J Med 1992;327:1899-905.
36. Shapiro S. Case-control surveillance. In: Strom BL, ed. Pharmacoepidemiology, 2nd ed. Chichester: Wiley, 1994: 301-22.
37. Alter MJ, Mares A, Hadler SC, Maynard JE. The effect of underreporting on the apparent incidence and epidemiology of acute viral hepatitis. Am J Epidemiol 1987;125: 133-9.
38. Kleinman S, Alter H, Busch M, et al. Increased detection of hepatitis C virus (HCV)-infected blood donors by a multiple-antigen HCV enzyme immunoassay. Transfusion 1992;32:805-13.
39. Busch MP, Korelitz JJ, Kleinman SH, et al. Declining value of alanine aminotransferase in screening of blood donors to prevent posttransfusion hepatitis B and C virus infection. Transfusion 1995;35:903-10.
40. Fisher LD, van Belle G. Biostatistics: A methodology for the health sciences. New York: Wiley, 1993.
41. Kramer MS. Clinical epidemiology and biostatistics. Berlin: Springer-Verlag, 1988.
42. Snedecor GW, Cochran WG. Statistical methods. Ames: The Iowa State University Press, 1967.
43. Angell M. The ethics of clinical research in the third world. N Engl J Med 1997;337:847-9.
44. Varmus H, Satcher D. Ethical complexities of conducting research in developing countries. N Engl J Med 1997; 337:1003-5.

In: Brecher ME, Busch MP, eds.
Research Design and Analysis
Bethesda, MD: American Association of Blood Banks, 1998

2

Meta-Analysis and Study Design

Eleftherios C. Vamvakas, MD, MPhil, PhD, MPH, MPA

META-ANALYSIS (OR STATISTICAL OVERVIEW) is the structured and systematic integration of information from different studies of a given problem.[1] It refers to the *disciplined* synthesis of previous research findings where the results of multiple reports on the efficacy of an intervention are compared, contrasted, and reanalyzed. When these results are discrepant, or if the variation among the reported findings is too great to be attributed to chance, the purpose of the statistical overview is to investigate the reasons for the disagreements between the studies. When the available results are concordant, the goal of the meta-analysis is to derive, through the application of a number of quantitative techniques, a measure of the effect of the intervention *across* the combined reports. This measure is referred to as the "average" or "summary" effect of the treatment under study.[1-6]

This chapter describes how meta-analysis is used, outlines the component parts of a meta-analysis, presents the reasons why statistical overviews undertaken to establish the existence of a treatment effect should combine only results obtained from randomized controlled trials (RCTs) (as op-

Eleftherios C. Vamvakas, MD, MPhil, PhD, MPH, MPA, Chief, Pathology and Laboratory Medicine Service, New York VA Medical Center, Attending Pathologist, New York University Medical Center, and Associate Professor of Pathology, New York University School of Medicine, New York, New York

posed to observational studies), and discusses criteria for assessing the quality of completed RCTs for inclusion in a meta-analysis. Research on the relationship between the transfusion of leukocyte-containing blood components and postoperative bacterial infection will be used throughout the text as an example to illustrate these concepts.

The Use of Meta-Analysis

Meta-analysis differs from the traditional, narrative reviews of the literature in which the author attempts to compare and interpret diverse studies within a particular research domain. With the traditional approach, the author summarizes study outcomes as positive, neutral, or negative, and then completes what is often called a "vote count" by summing the number of studies that reported each type of outcome. Meta-analysis differs from these "qualitative" reviews of the literature in that: 1) *All* completed investigations that meet specific eligibility criteria are retrieved and included in the overview; 2) The degree of agreement among the studies is evaluated based on statistical criteria, and the synthesis of the findings proceeds *only* if the variation in the reported results is small enough to be attributed to chance; and 3) Providing that this prerequisite is met, *quantitative* methods are used to calculate the "average" effect of the intervention and to test that effect for statistical significance.[1-6] If a meta-analysis is conducted in accordance with these guidelines,[2,7-10] the reader can benefit from "an objective view of the research literature, unaffected by the sometimes distorting lens of individual experience and personal preference that can affect a less structured review."[11(p246)]

Meta-analyses generate some general conclusion about the efficacy of an intervention. Statistical overviews are a supplement, not an alternative, to RCTs, which remain the gold standard for evaluating the efficacy of medical interventions[12] but need to be supplemented by meta-analyses in order to broaden the applicability of the findings. RCTs usually use restricted eligibility criteria for patient enrollment, in an effort to enhance the power of the trial to detect a treatment effect. A homogeneous patient population makes it easier to attribute any observed differences in outcome between the treatment and the control groups to the effect of the intervention under study, rather than to baseline differences in the characteristics of the patients enrolled in each group. RCTs that enroll homogeneous patient populations can detect a treatment effect with a smaller number of patients, as compared with studies that use unselected subjects. The increase in study power comes at the expense of a decrease in the applicability (or generalizability) of the findings of the RCT. If a study uses restrictive criteria for patient enrollment, the results of this RCT may apply only to a similarly selected population of patients.[13]

A meta-analysis integrates the findings of separate studies, which usually differ in many aspects of their design. This variability in the design attributes of reports included in a meta-analysis results in greater generalizability of the finding of a statistical overview, as compared with the result of an RCT. By combining studies with disparate design characteristics, meta-analysis permits the examination of the effect of an intervention in many different situations. If the effect is consistent in all studies, this consistency favors a true treatment effect, rather than one due to chance or some systematic error or bias that compromised the results of all completed investigations. As stated by Hennekens, "the most persuasive evidence to support a judgment of a cause-[and]-effect relationship arises when a number of studies, conducted by different investigators at various times using alternative methodology in a variety of geographic and cultural settings and among different populations, all show similar results."[14(p41)]

There is consensus among epidemiologists on the appropriate sequence of steps that need to be followed when a meta-analysis is conducted (Table 2-1). The experts agree that meta-analyses should be limited to RCTs. If both RCTs and observational studies on the effect of an intervention are to be considered in an overview, the findings of observational studies should be integrated separately from the results of RCTs.[15-17] However, the experts disagree on other quality criteria to be used for disqualifying studies from inclusion in a meta-analysis. They also disagree whether *any* randomized trial, no matter how poorly designed and executed, should ever be excluded from a statistical overview.[18] The second step in the sequence shown in Table 2-1 (ie, the *selection* of

Table 2-1. Sequence of Steps To Be Followed in Conducting a Meta-Analysis

1. Retrieval of all completed studies on the effect of the intervention of interest.
2. Determination of the eligibility of the retrieved studies for inclusion in the analysis, based on criteria specified in advance and relating to:
   * the scope of the hypothesis under study
   * the quality of the retrieved studies
3. Extraction of data from each study on the effect of the intervention of interest.
4. Assessment of the degree of concordance between the studies (both conceptually and using statistical criteria).
5. If the studies are concordant, calculation of a "summary" or "average" estimate of the effect of the intervention across the combined investigations.
6. If the studies are discordant, examination of the reasons for the disagreements between the studies.

---

studies for inclusion in an overview) remains a highly contested area in the field of meta-analysis.

Whether studies should be selected for inclusion in an overview based on explicit quality criteria depends on our conceptions of the proper role, scope, and meaning of meta-analysis in general, and the stated purpose of a given overview in particular. When the purpose of the synthesis of previous research findings is to provide an estimate of the most likely magnitude of a treatment effect, so that the investigators can design a definitive RCT that will enroll as many patients as are needed for establishing the existence of the effect of the intervention, it is probably adequate to rely on the totality of the evidence and to include all completed studies in the overview regardless of their quality. This statistical exercise should be part of the planning phase of any RCT, and it is not usually intended for publication as an original report; accordingly, the time and effort required for an assessment of the quality of the completed studies may not be justified. However, if the purpose of the meta-analysis is to reach a conclusion about the existence of a treatment effect by combining data on patient populations enrolled in separate studies, the quality of the studies to be included in the overview should be explicitly addressed in the report of the meta-analysis. If it is not, the overview may be criticized[19,20] as an "exercise in megasilliness" where "a mass of reports—good, bad, and indifferent—are fed into the computer in the hope that people will cease caring about the quality of the material on which the conclusions are based" and where "garbage in, garbage out, a well-known axiom of computer specialists, applies with equal force."[19(p517)]

Jenicek,[1] O'Rourke and Detsky,[21] and Goodman[11] have proposed that the assessment of the quality of the completed studies on the effect of an intervention should be the *primary* purpose (or one of the main reasons) for conducting a meta-analysis. According to Jenicek,[1] the first phase of a statistical overview must be a "qualitative" meta-analysis, which must precede the "quantitative" phase of the report. An assessment of the quality of the retrieved studies must be made, and studies of unacceptable quality must be rejected. O'Rourke and Detsky[21] assert that the major contribution of a meta-analysis lies in the attention it draws to flaws in the design and conduct of previous studies. When all published studies are subjected to a detailed review of the methods—with a focus on the impact of the methods on the validity of the results—inadequacies can be identified, and their resolution can be encouraged. Recognized shortcomings can be avoided in future individual research efforts, so that more valid results are produced.[21] In Goodman's words, a meta-analysis should "raise research and editorial standards, by calling attention to the strengths and weaknesses of the body of research in an area."[11(pp245-6)]

Component Parts of a Meta-Analysis

A meta-analysis proceeds in a strict sequence of retrieval of eligible studies and data extraction, assessment of the degree of concordance between the reports, and either the examination of the reasons for the disagreements between the studies or the combination of the results of the individual investigations where indicated. In the end, findings from studies with varying design attributes are often integrated, but it is important to remember that a meta-analysis "pools" the treatment effects calculated from individual studies and not the data on the individual patients enrolled in each report. The treatment effect for each trial included in the overview is based exclusively on the outcomes of the treated patients and the controls who participated in that study.

An overview by the fixed-effects method combines a series of 2×2 tables (Table 2-2), as though these represented strata of patients enrolled in the same study. The findings from individual strata are combined, according each stratum a weight commensurate with its sample size.[5,6,22,23] In this process, it is assumed that there is a uniform (or "fixed") treatment effect in all of the studies included in the meta-analysis. Studies are thought to have generated different estimates of that fixed effect solely because of the play of chance, that is, because of random sampling variation from study to study. This is a reasonable assumption to make *if* the design attributes of the combined studies are similar, and they permit an expectation that the treatment will have the same effect in all of the studies.

When the combined studies differ with respect to important design attributes, it is not possible to assume that all the studies measure the same (or "fixed") treatment effect. For example, studies of the relationship between perioperative

Table 2-2. 2×2 Contingency Table Counts From Randomized Controlled Trials of the Relationship Between Perioperative Allogeneic Blood Transfusion and Postoperative Bacterial Infection

	Postoperative Infection	
	Yes	No
Treatment group (patients prospectively randomized to receive allogeneic blood)	a	b
Control group (patients prospectively randomized to receive autologous or filtered allogeneic blood)	c	d

Odds ratio = $\dfrac{a \times d}{b \times c}$

allogeneic blood transfusion and postoperative bacterial infection[24-35] have differed with regard to important aspects of their design, and these differences (Table 2-3) make it reasonable to assume that the effect of perioperative blood transfusion should have varied among the completed investigations. A meta-analysis by the random-effects method[18,23] is advocated for these circumstances where the combined reports differ from each other in complex ways. In this setting, an assumption is made that varying treatment effects, calculated by individual studies, are randomly positioned around a central value, that is, around the summary or average effect of the intervention under study.

Regardless of whether a fixed- or a random-effects method is used for the analysis, results from separate studies can be combined *only* when the estimates of the treatment effect(s) are sufficiently close to one another and all differences in the reported findings can be attributed to chance.[1-6,36-38] This fundamental prerequisite is referred to as "homogeneity of effects." Statistical techniques are not to be used to integrate apples and oranges, that is, contradictory findings from studies that have reported heterogeneous effects of an intervention. Statistical reviewers of the Food and Drug Administration have denigrated, as mere computational exercises, all meta-analyses that had combined study reports

Table 2-3. Differences in Design Attributes of Randomized Controlled Trials Investigating the Relationship Between Perioperative Allogeneic Blood Transfusion and Postoperative Bacterial Infection

1. Patient population enrolled (patients undergoing elective colorectal cancer surgery vs patients undergoing colorectal cancer resection).
2. Frequency of risk factors for postoperative infection in enrolled patients.
3. Single-center vs multicenter study design.
4. Type of red cell product given to the treatment group (allogeneic whole blood vs buffy-coat-poor allogeneic red cells).
5. Type of red cell product given to the control group (autologous red cells or whole blood vs filtered allogeneic red cells or whole blood).
6. Criteria used for the diagnosis of postoperative infection.

in the presence of unexplained heterogeneity.[36-38] Instead of pooling heterogeneous findings, authors of overviews should provide an analysis of the possible reasons for the noted disagreements among the completed investigations.[1,2,11]

Figure 2-1 shows the 95% confidence interval (CI) for the relative risk (RR) of postoperative bacterial infection in patients receiving perioperative allogeneic blood transfusion, as compared with the recipients of autologous or filtered blood components. Five RCTs[29-34] investigated the hypothesis of an increased risk of infection in the allogeneic transfusion group among patients undergoing elective colorectal cancer resection, and they produced an RR of infection in association with allogeneic blood transfusion that varied from 0.9[30,31,33] to 6.5.[29] The associated 95% CIs extended between 0.6[28,29,31] and 33.1,[27] indicating marked heterogeneity. This degree of discrepancy in the findings of the studies precludes

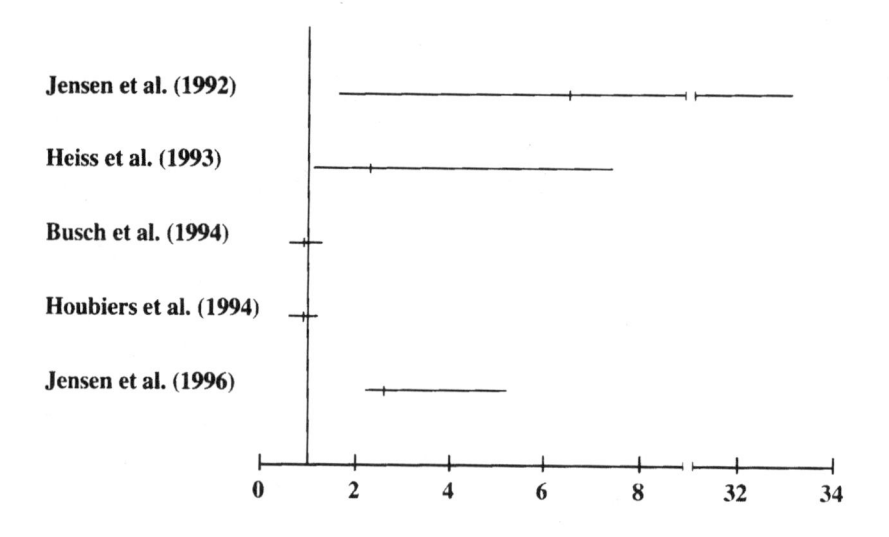

Figure 2-1. Heterogeneity of effects across the studies of Jensen et al,[29] Heiss et al,[32] Busch et al,[30,31] Houbiers et al,[33] and Jensen et al,[34] which evaluated the relationship between perioperative allogeneic blood transfusion and postoperative bacterial infection. The relative risk (RR) of postoperative infection in recipients of allogeneic (as compared with autologous or filtered) blood components is plotted on a linear scale, along with the associated 95% confidence interval (CI) for the RR. An RR of 1 indicates no transfusion effect. When the 95% CI extends on both sides of the null value, the reported transfusion effect is not statistically significant.

the calculation of a summary or average transfusion effect across the published RCTs.

Rationale for Restricting Meta-Analyses to Randomized Controlled Trials

When two medical events are associated, there may be a number of possible explanations for this relationship.[39,40] The association may be a causal one and differences in the treatment received may be responsible for differences in the observed outcome. On the other hand, the association may not be a causal one and could be due to confounding factors or bias. Confounding refers to the situation where an unrecognized variable is associated with *both* the outcome of interest *and* its putative cause. Bias is any systematic error in the design of a study (or execution of the study protocol) that may result in a systematic deviation from the truth when the data are analyzed and reported.[41] Selection (allocation) bias refers to systematic differences between patients who receive a particular treatment and those who do not if these differences are the result of a judgment on the part of the investigators as to who might benefit from (and should preferentially receive) the treatment under study. Observation (ascertainment) bias refers to systematic differences in the diagnosis by the investigators of subsequent disease in patients who received the treatment and those who did not.

Limitations of Observational Studies

In prospective or retrospective observational studies of the relationship between perioperative blood transfusion and postoperative bacterial infection, there is a selection bias in the allocation of the treatment under study (allogeneic red cell transfusion) to *sicker* patients with low hemoglobin, compromised cardiopulmonary status, etc, who are also the subset of patients most likely to develop postoperative infection.[26,28] In a similar vein, there are baseline differences between the groups of transfused and untransfused patients in a number of variables pertaining to the factors that generate the need for transfusion in one of the groups. Many of these variables are also associated with the risk of postoperative septic complications[26,28,35] and may function as confounding factors of the relationship between transfusion and postoperative infection. In addition, when these studies are reviewed, a question is raised whether the criteria for the diagnosis of postoperative infection may have been applied differentially to transfused and untransfused patients by investigators who were aware of the transfusion status of each patient. In making diagnoses of infection, these authors may have been influenced by their own conscious or subconscious beliefs about the existence of an adverse transfusion effect.

More specifically, Table 2-4 lists the variables that are associated with postoperative septic complications in the setting of elective colorectal cancer resection.[26,28,35] Many of these factors are associated with a need for perioperative transfusion as well,[35,42,43] and they may confound the association of transfusion with postoperative infection. As an example of one of these potential confounding factors, which applies to the relationship between perioperative transfusion and postoperative urinary tract infection (UTI), Fig 2-2 shows the effect of the number of days with indwelling urinary catheter on postoperative UTI. This variable is the predominant risk factor for nosocomial UTI. Urinary catheters are implicated in 80% of nosocomial UTIs in the United States.[44] Transfused patients have indwelling urinary catheters for a longer period of time than untransfused patients. In a study of 492 patients undergoing colorectal cancer resection,[35] the 75th and the 95th percentiles for the number of days with indwelling urinary catheter were 7 and 14 days, respectively, in the transfused group, as compared with 4.5 and 7.5 days, respectively, in the untransfused group (p<0.0001). Similarly, the 75th and the 95th percentiles were 7 and 17 days, respectively, in patients who developed postoperative infection, as compared with 4.5 and 8.5 days, respectively, in patients who did not develop an infection (p<0.0001). In this study,[35] the number of days with indwelling urinary catheter was the most highly significant predictor of postoperative UTI in a multivariate analysis that also considered gender, presence of chronic systemic illness, leukopenia on admission, duration of anesthesia, perioperative blood loss, and perioperative allogeneic blood transfusion as potential predictors of UTI.

Table 2-4. Factors Potentially Associated With Postoperative Septic Complications in Patients Undergoing Elective Colorectal Cancer Resection*

I. Risk factors for postoperative infection at any site
   1. Chronic systemic illness (eg, malnutrition, congestive heart, lung, kidney, or liver failure, etc)
   2. American Society of Anesthesiologists class of the patient
   3. Preoperative or intraoperative irradiation/chemotherapy
   4. Preoperative or intraoperative immunosuppression
   5. Prophylactic perioperative administration of antibiotics
   6. Pre-existing infection
   7. Preoperative anemia or leukopenia
   8. Dukes' stage and histologic differentiation of the tumor and tumor location
   9. Type of operation (ie, colectomy or anterior resection vs abdomino-perineal resection)
   10. Experience and qualifications of the surgeon
   11. Duration of anesthesia
   12. Anesthetic agent used
   13. Intraoperative blood loss and lowest recorded diastolic and systolic blood pressure during surgery
II. Risk factors for wound infection
   1. Drainage of the area of operation
   2. Colostomy
   3. Wound left open without colostomy
   4. Fecal contamination of the operative site
   5. Intraoperative endoscopy
   6. Re-operation during the same hospitalization for a reason other than wound infection
III. Risk factors for pneumonia
   1. Period of impaired consciousness/strong sedation preceding a diagnosis of pneumonia
   2. Intubation preceding a diagnosis of pneumonia
   3. Gastric acid neutralization therapy
IV. Risk factors for urinary tract infection
   1. Number of days with indwelling urinary catheter preceding a diagnosis of urinary tract infection
V. Risk factors for bacteremia
   1. Number of days with indwelling central vascular or peripheral vascular or femoral catheters preceding a diagnosis of bacteremia

*Modified from Vamvakas and Blajchman.[26]

**Days with indwelling
urinary catheter**

Transfusion – – – – – ? – – – – ▶ Urinary tract infection

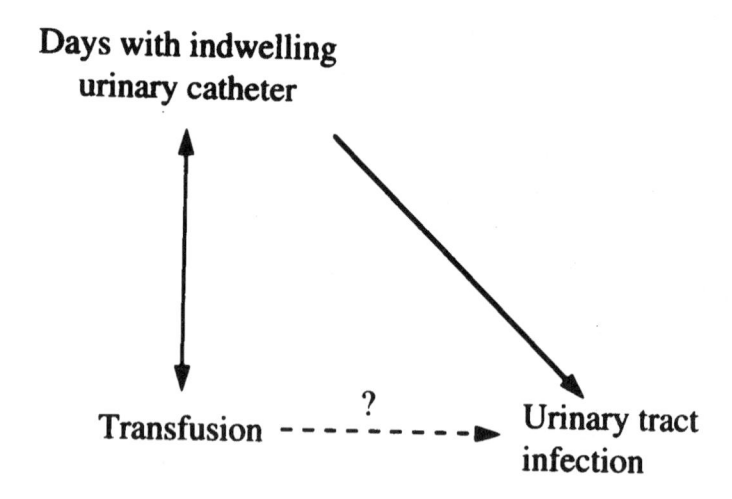

Figure 2-2. Confounding effect of the number of days with indwelling urinary catheter on the relationship between perioperative transfusion and postoperative urinary tract infection (UTI). The longer a patient has an indwelling urinary catheter the greater the risk of postoperative UTI. (The solid straight line in the figure indicates that the number of days with indwelling urinary catheter is an established risk factor for UTI.[44]) Transfused patients have indwelling urinary catheters for a longer period of time than untransfused patients when they undergo colorectal cancer resection.[35] Any observed association between perioperative transfusion and postoperative UTI in the setting of colorectal cancer resection may be due to the relationship between the number of days with indwelling urinary catheter and *both* perioperative transfusion *and* postoperative UTI.

Because the risk of UTI depends on the length of time that a patient has an indwelling urinary catheter, and the transfused patients have indwelling urinary catheters for a longer period of time than the untransfused patients, perioperative blood transfusion is bound to be associated with postoperative UTI because of its association with this confounding factor, that is, the number of days with indwelling urinary catheter. It is possible that transfusion may also have an *independent* effect on postoperative UTI, which is due to the transfusion per se, as opposed to the association of transfusion with the confounding factor. To establish the existence of any such independent effect, investigators must adjust for the effect of the number of days with indwelling urinary catheter, as well as the effects of gender, presence of chronic systemic illness, and other risk factors for postoperative

UTI.[35] If the effects of these confounding factors are held constant, the effect of transfusion on postoperative UTI can be separated from the effects of the other variables, and any residual association between transfusion and UTI can potentially be ascribed to the transfusion per se.

Observational studies adjust for the effects of confounding factors by the use of statistical techniques.[45] Known and measurable variables, identified by the investigators in the design phase of a study[46] and measured in the course of the study, are introduced into multivariate regression models that separate the effects of these variables from the effect of transfusion. Factors such as the difficulty of the operation, the skill of the surgeon, and the nutritional and overall health status of the patient are potential confounding factors (because they are probably associated with both perioperative transfusion and postoperative infection), but they cannot be precisely quantified and they are difficult to control by statistical techniques. Because the tools available to the authors of observational studies cannot adjust for the effects of *all* the variables that confound an association under study, it is not possible to establish a causal relationship by the use of an observational study design.[14,39,40]

Meta-Analyses of Randomized Controlled Trials vs Meta-Analyses of Observational Studies

As discussed previously, RCTs are prospective clinical experiments in which patients who have agreed to participate in a study are *randomly* allocated by the investigators to treatment and control groups that do, and do not, receive the intervention under study.[47] RCTs are considered to be the most powerful method of investigation in clinical research[48] because—if they are correctly conducted—they can eliminate bias[41] and they can also considerably reduce (or eliminate) confounding factors[14] as alternative explanations for any noted differences in outcome between patients who have or have not received a particular treatment.[47]

More specifically, if randomization is used, neither the investigator nor the participant can influence the allocation of the patient to the treatment or the control group because neither one of them knows what the assignment will be prior to the patient's decision to enter the study. Also, providing that the RCT is designed as a double-blind study, preconceived notions about the benefit from the treatment cannot influence the reporting of signs and symptoms by the patient or the assessment of disease activity by the investigator. Finally, thanks to the play of chance, randomization should produce groups that are balanced with regard to the level of all known and unknown confounding variables of the association under study, so that differences in outcome between the treatment and the control groups cannot be traced to differences in the level of confounding factors between the arms of the trial.[47]

In RCTs that study the relationship between perioperative allogeneic blood transfusion and postoperative bacterial infection,[29-34] the process of random assignment of subjects to groups would be expected to produce treatment and control groups with the same baseline need for transfusion and risk of infection if the randomization procedure were correctly implemented. With this caveat, the contingency table counts from each RCT (ie, the counts a, b, c, and d in Table 2-2) should be free from the effects of both confounding factors and selection bias. The odds ratio ad/bc (the RR of postoperative infection between the treatment and the control groups) should reflect the true deleterious effect of allogeneic transfusion, establishing a cause-and-effect relationship if one exists.[14] Providing that the contingency table counts are indeed free from the effect of confounding variables, such a simple, univariate analysis is sufficient for the calculation of the RR in RCTs.

In observational studies of the same association,[35] patients are passively observed by the investigators as they undergo perioperative transfusion, and transfused and untransfused patients differ with respect to known and unknown determinants of the need for transfusion and the risk of infection. As already stated, the authors of original observational reports used multivariate regression analysis to control for the effects of known and measurable confounding variables.[12,45,46] Contingency table counts that are extracted from the reports of observational studies for use in statistical overviews (Table 2-5) have not been subjected to multivariate analysis by either the authors of the observational reports or the meta-analysts, and—indeed—they have not undergone any manipulation for adjusting for the effects of confounding fac-

Table 2-5. 2×2 Contingency Table Counts from Observational Studies of the Relationship Between Perioperative Blood Transfusion and Postoperative Bacterial Infection

	Postoperative Infection	
	Yes	No
Treatment group (transfused patients)	a	b
Control group (untransfused patients)	c	d

Odds ratio $= \dfrac{a \times d}{b \times c}$

tors. The odds ratio (RR, ad/bc) that is calculated from a simple, univariate analysis of a contingency table extracted from an observational study is far more tainted by the effects of confounding factors than are the results of the original observational reports as published by the primary investigators. However, meta-analyses of observational studies (such as the reported overviews of investigations of the relationship between perioperative allogeneic blood transfusion and cancer recurrence[49-52]) extract 2×2 contingency table counts from each study, use these four counts to calculate an RR for the corresponding report, and then combine the series of 2×2 contingency table counts without taking into account the effects of the confounding variables that are incorporated in these unadjusted results.

For this reason, only results from RCTs can be integrated when the purpose of a meta-analysis is to investigate the existence of a causal relationship.[9,18,21] Observational studies produce larger estimates of a treatment effect compared to randomized trials because of the effects of uncontrolled confounding factors and selection bias.[53-55] Accordingly, to prevent the calculation of an inflated average treatment effect, observational studies investigating the hypothesis considered by an overview must be either analyzed separately or excluded from the meta-analysis altogether. However, two-thirds of the overviews published between 1982 and 1989 were based on observational studies.[56]

Assessment of the Quality of Randomized Controlled Trials for Inclusion in a Meta-Analysis

A study may be reported in a scientific journal, but publication is in no way an endorsement of its results or conclusions.[57] Important limitations in the design, conduct, and analysis of an RCT may not be detected by the peer-review process,[58] and there have been many reports of errors or unsubstantiated conclusions reached by trials published in medical journals.[59-62] Readers must develop the skills necessary to critically assess all reports of clinical research and to decide how to make the best use of the findings.

A randomized design does not exclude the possibilities of selection bias, observation bias, and confounding by known and unknown cofounders. Any system of randomization can be tampered with and compromised, and enrolled patients and investigators can become aware of the next treatment assignment.[63,64] Inadequate concealment of the next treatment allocation can lead to bias in many ways, sometimes as the result of deliberate subversions, sometimes as the result of subconscious actions. If those responsible for admitting patients into the RCT have foreknowledge of the treatment allocations, they may channel subjects with a better prognosis to the treatment group, and those with a poorer prognosis to the control group, or vice versa. That could easily be accomplished by delaying a patient's entry into the study until the next desired allocation appears, by excluding eligible participants from the trial, or encouraging them to refuse entry.

Unblinded or single-blind RCTs can be compromised by observation bias as much as the prospective observational studies of the same hypothesis because there is no difference between the unblinded RCTs and the prospective observational studies in the way the outcome of interest is ascertained in both treated patients and controls. Randomization does *not* guard against the effect of preconceived notions regarding benefit from a treatment on the part of either patients or investigators. Blinding is not part of the definition of a randomized controlled design, and observation bias can often be responsible for the findings of published, unblinded RCTs.

Finally, while probability theory dictates that randomization should produce balanced comparison groups in RCTs that enroll *infinitely large* patient populations, the random assignment of subjects to groups does not guarantee balance in the levels of the confounding factors present in the arms of any ordinary trial with a finite sample size. Failure of randomization to equally distribute all confounding variables between the arms of an RCT is a major concern in small studies,[65] but it can also occur in very large investigations because of sheer "bad luck." Differences between the treatment and the control groups in important patient characteristics are possible in any RCT, and—when present—they can generate highly misleading conclusions. For this reason, unless the RCT enrolls an exceptionally large patient population,[66] the success of randomization needs to be monitored by measuring all known confounding factors on the enrolled patients and by comparing the distribution of those variables between the prospectively formed arms of the study. Like the authors of observational studies, the authors of RCTs should report the levels of all known confounding variables in the comparison groups of their trial.

In summary, investigators need to provide sufficient detail about their randomization procedure and blinding technique, as well as the levels of all known confounding factors in the arms of their study, for readers to assess the validity of the conclusions reached by an RCT. If this information is not provided, or if the procedures used do not ensure freedom of the results from selection bias, observation bias, and effects of confounding factors, a cause-and-effect relationship is not established, and the findings of the RCT are subject to alternative explanations. These potential limitations of the individual RCTs are an important argument for conducting meta-analyses of trials to supplement the available RCTs. The result of no single RCT can be considered definitive without supporting evidence. Meta-analyses of trials can aid in the interpretation of the results of RCTs by investigating the *consistency* of the findings of all available randomized studies, as well as the consistency of these results with data from laboratory, animal, epidemiologic, and other clinical research. Meta-analyses can also grade and rank the quality of the completed studies, so that any judgment regarding the efficacy of a medical intervention can be based on investigations of high scientific validity.

Threats to the Validity of the Results of Randomized Controlled Trials

The assessment of the quality of studies retrieved from the literature has been listed as a necessary part of any statistical overview in the early guidelines for meta-analysis in clinical research.[1,2,11] This position was also endorsed by Moher and Olkin in their call for standards for publishing reports of meta-analyses.[7] Formal instruments for evaluating the quality of completed RCTs have been developed.[67-69] Chalmers et al[67] reported a detailed list of the items to be used for scoring the quality of published RCTs on a scale from 0 to 1. Detsky et al[68] presented a simplified scale, and Zelen[69] proposed a third instrument. Lichtenstein et al[70] and Feinstein[71] presented guidelines for evaluating observational studies.

Liberati et al[72] used the instrument of Chalmers et al[67] in a formal grading of 63 RCTs of primary treatment for breast cancer. The average quality score was 0.50 (95% CI, 0.46-0.54). Telephone calls to the principal investigator improved the quality scores by an average of 0.07, indicating that some of the deficiencies lay in reporting rather than performance.[69] Guidelines for the reporting of RCTs have been presented.[73-76]

Disagreements between trials are frequently noted in medical research, and the variation in the quality of the completed RCTs can sometimes explain the variation in the reported findings. Figure 2-1 illustrates the magnitude of the disagreements among the RCTs regarding the relationship between perioperative allogeneic blood transfusion and postoperative bacterial infection in patients having elective colorectal cancer resection. As reported, the results of those RCTs suggested a 1100%-difference in the magnitude of the postulated adverse transfusion effect; that effect varied from a 10% reduction (p>0.25) to an 11-fold increase (p<0.001) in the risk of postoperative bacterial infection. In Fig 2-1, the findings of Jensen et al[29,34] are shown not as published, but as recalculated according to the intention-to-treat principle.[77-80] Even after this correction, the adverse transfusion effect varies from a 10% reduction to a 6.5-fold increase in the risk of infection. Biologic reasons for this variation (Table 2-3) have been discussed,[26] and Table 2-6 lists four methodologic reasons that might potentially further account for a portion of

Table 2-6. Possible Threats to the Internal Validity of the Findings of Randomized Controlled Trials of the Relationship Between Perioperative Allogeneic Blood Transfusion and Postoperative Bacterial Infection

1. Selection bias in the allocation of the enrolled patients to allogeneic vs autologous/filtered allogeneic transfusion groups. (Were the investigators and the patients aware of the next treatment assigmnent prior to a patient's decision to enter the study?)
2. Observation bias in the ascertainment of the occurrence of postoperative infection. (Was the study unblinded or single-blind?)
3. Unbalanced distribution of known and unknown confounding factors between the allogeneic and autologous/filtered allogeneic transfusion groups. (Were all known confounding variables of the association under study measured in the course of the trial? Did the groups differ in terms of any of the patient characteristics listed in Table 2-4?)
4. Statistical analysis that does not serve the purpose of randomization. (Were any postrandomization patient withdrawals permitted? Were the stated conclusions based on an on-treatment [as opposed to intention-to-treat] comparison? Were the stated conclusions based on subgroup analyses rather than an overall comparison?)

---

this variation. Table 2-7 presents an evaluation of four of the studies[29-33] by a meta-analysis.[28] The issues relating to the possible methodologic limitations of published RCTs (Table 2-6)[47,81] are further discussed below.

The random assignment of subjects to groups is expected to both generate an unpredictable assignment sequence and to ensure concealment of this sequence until each enrolled patient is allocated to either the treatment or the control group of an RCT. Schultz et al[81] evaluated the adequacy of the measures taken in 250 RCTs to ensure concealment of the allocation sequence. They considered that central randomization, coded bottles of drugs or drugs prepared by a pharmacy, as well as serially numbered, opaque, sealed envelopes, were adequate measures to ensure concealment. Other approaches, such as alternation of or reference to case record numbers or dates of birth, were considered to be inadequate in this regard. The authors[81] observed that, following adjustment for other aspects of RCT quality (ie, blinded design, inclusion of all randomized patients in the analysis), studies in

Table 2-7. Quality Scores of Unblinded Randomized Controlled Trials of the Effect of Allogeneic Blood Transfusion on Postoperative Bacterial Infection in Elective Colorectal Cancer Surgery*

Criterion	Jensen et al[29]	Busch et al[30,31]	Heiss et al[32]	Houbiers et al[33]
1. Enrollment limited to patients with colorectal cancer	0	0.2	0.2	0.2
2. Enrollment limited to patients undergoing elective surgery	0.2	0.2	0.2	0.2
3. Postrandomization exclusions of patients not permitted	0	0	0.2	0
4. Analysis according to the "intention-to-treat" principle presented	0	0.2	0.2	0.2
5. Sufficient proof provided that the purpose of randomization to equally distribute confounding factors between the groups was achieved	0	0.2	0.2	0.2
Total quality score	0.2	0.8	1.00	0.8

*From Vamvakas EC.[82] Based on the reports of these RCTs, the postoperative diagnoses of infection were made by unblinded investigators in all the studies. For a discussion of the selection of the quality criteria used for the evaluation of these RCTs see Vamvakas.[28] Based on the criteria shown above, the median quality score for the four studies[30-33] included in the meta-analysis[28] was 0.8.

which concealment had been inadequate yielded larger estimates of the treatment effect (p<0.001), exaggerating the effect of an intervention by 41% on average as compared with trials in which the investigators had adequately concealed the treatment allocation.

Trials that were not double-blind also produced larger estimates of treatment effects (p=0.01), exaggerating those effects by 17% compared with blinded investigations. Schultz et al[81] had anticipated that the lack of double-blinding would have inflated the calculated treatment effects by more than 17%, and they commented that "trials that reported double-blinding usually provided little, if any, information on the method used. Thus, some trials claiming to be double-blind may not have been, and so misclassification error could have caused an underestimate of the independent effect of not double-blinding."[81(p412)] Other investigators have also reported that trials called double-blind are not always double-blind[83] or that they may become unblinded.[84,85]

Reports of exaggerated treatment effects can also be due to an unbalanced distribution of confounding variables between the arms of an RCT.[47] For example, studies that reported an unusually large adverse effect of perioperative allogeneic transfusion on postoperative bacterial infection (Fig 2-1) may have included a disproportionate number of patients with risk factors for postoperative infection in the treatment group, as compared with the control group. Studies that did not detect an adverse transfusion effect may have included fewer patients with such factors in the treatment group compared with the control group. The published reports of some of the trials listed in Fig 2-1[29,34] did not provide adequate information on the distribution of confounding factors in the treatment and control groups of the studies,[28] leaving the reported findings subject to this alternative explanation.

To reap the benefits conferred by randomization (ie, to achieve equal distribution of all confounding factors between the comparison groups of a trial), investigators must conduct an "intention-to-treat" analysis, and they must compare the *entire* groups of patients that are formed by the random assignment of subjects to groups.[77-80] No withdrawals of patients should be allowed after the randomization step, and all patients should be analyzed within the groups to which they were randomly assigned, no matter how much or how little treatment they actually received.[14,47] Subgroup analyses should be clearly identified as such, and they should be considered as hypothesis-generating rather than as hypothesis-testing. Confounding variables cannot be presumed to be evenly balanced between patient *sub*groups created in the analysis phase of an RCT.

In an "on-treatment" analysis, the analysis is restricted to patients who did receive the treatment that they were expected to receive according to the randomization scheme.[86] For the purposes of causal inference, this comparison is valid only if the withdrawn subjects have been excluded in a random fashion. If the exclusions have been dictated by factors related to the treatment and the outcome under study, any on-treatment analysis may be seriously biased,[79] and it should be considered equivalent to the comparisons made in observational studies.[14,47,77-80] For example, if untransfused subjects are excluded from the analysis of an RCT investigating the relationship between allogeneic blood transfusion and postoperative bacterial infection (Table 2-2), the withdrawals are based on each patient's need for transfusion. An argument that these exclusions do not have an impact on the distribution of confounding factors between the groups (eg, the patient's physical status and severity of illness, the surgeon's skill, the difficulty of the operation, etc) might be entertained only if it could be supported by a most detailed comparison of the remaining subjects on all known confounding variables.

Selection of Studies for Inclusion in a Meta-Analysis

After the quality of all retrieved studies has been considered by the meta-analysts, and quality scores have been assigned to the studies based on an instrument created or selected for this purpose, poor-quality reports are usually excluded from an overview. RCTs are retained for analysis if they have achieved a quality score that exceeds the mean or median quality score for all studies available from the literature, or if they exceed a minimum quality score arbitrarily set by the meta-analysts for the particular overview. For example, Vamvakas[28] excluded the trial of Jensen et al[29] from a meta-analysis of the RCTs of perioperative allogeneic blood transfusion and postoperative bacterial infection published prior to 1995, because the quality score attained by the trial of Jensen et al[29] was below the median quality score for the studies available at the time of the overview (Table 2-7).

If studies of inferior quality are to be retained in the analysis, the investigations can be stratified by quality score, and summary estimates of the treatment effect can be calculated separately for each stratum of quality. If the treatment effects differ across the strata, the average effect calculated from studies of superior quality can be considered to be the valid one.[87] Another approach calls for incorporating the quality score of each report into the weight assigned to that study, and for weighting the summary effect of an intervention to reflect more heavily the findings of RCTs of high scientific validity than the results of poor-quality studies.[88] Methods currently used by meta-analysts[3-6] weigh each component study according to its sample size. However, there is general agreement that, if studies of poor quality are to be included in an overview, the differences in quality must be taken into account in the analysis.[66,87,89,90] Accordingly, methods for adjusting the weight of the studies to also incorporate the quality of each report are under development.

The main argument for including studies that are not of the best quality in a meta-analysis is that a larger number of studies permits examination of the effect of an intervention in more situations. For example, by excluding the study of Jensen et al,[29] Vamvakas[28] precluded examination of the effect of transfusion of unmodified red cell components, as all studies included in that meta-analysis had transfused buffy-coat-poor red cells to the treatment group. However, the advantage of considering the effect of a treatment in more situations must be balanced against the disadvantage of including potentially questionable results.

In summary, there is no single or best strategy for dealing with studies of inferior quality in conducting an overview, and all methods for selecting studies for inclusion in a meta-analysis are controversial. No matter what strategy is adopted, meta-analysts must describe this strategy and their reasons for choice of strategy. In addressing this problem, authors of overviews have to rely on their judgment because no approach is suitable for all situations.

Conclusion

Meta-analysis can be an important research tool for the systematic evaluation of the quality of studies and the disciplined investigation of the reasons for disagreements among reports. In the past, traditional, narrative reviews of the literature served these functions in a less formal manner. Meta-analyses are much better suited for these purposes because of their objective and quantitative nature.

Meta-analyses have also been used to establish the existence of a treatment effect in situations where multiple small RCTs have been conducted, but have not demonstrated a statistically significant effect perhaps because of their small sample size. The value of meta-analysis in combining patient populations enrolled in separate studies for the purpose of documenting the existence of a treatment effect has been questioned.[91-93] This recent scrutiny of the value of meta-analyses in the medical literature was in part provoked by three discordant reports[94-96] on the degree of agreement between overviews of small trials and subsequently conducted large RCTs.[97] Meta-analyses and large trials disagree 10-35% of the time, that is, more often than would be expected by chance.[94-96] Until the reasons for the disagreements are better understood, medical practitioners should not rely on meta-analyses for concluding that the existence of a treatment effect has been established. However, the controversy over this specific use of meta-analysis should not detract from the value of overviews in assessing the quality of completed studies and the reasons for disagreements among reports. As stated by Ioannidis et al,[97(p1093)] future meta-analyses will likely "find an important role in addressing potential sources of heterogeneity rather than always trying to fit a common estimate (of a treatment effect) among diverse studies." The development of quantitative methods for examining sources of heterogeneity is an active area of research. Formal assessments of the quality of completed studies can contribute to an investigation of the sources of heterogeneity, and they should be one of the main reasons for conducting meta-analyses in the future.

In conclusion, a statistical overview can identify errors and shortcomings in completed studies and can explain why trial results differ. Critics should recognize that, if it were not for meta-analysis, many of the deficiencies in the quality of published research would not have been identified.[38] Guidelines for the conduct of meta-analyses have been provided,[1-8] so that the two recurrent criticisms of the method—the garbage in, garbage out and the apples and oranges metaphors[19,20]—can be avoided. Meta-analyses are, and should be treated as, observational and retrospective original reports. Quantitative results from overviews (including p values and 95% CIs for the size of treatment effects) should be considered as hypothesis-generating rather than hypothesis-testing. A hypothesis formulated by a meta-analysis may or may not be corroborated when a "definitive" RCT is conducted. However, the limitations of the reported research and the reasons for disagreements among the studies, as identified by a meta-analysis, can guide the design and the conduct of this "definitive" RCT in the future. Meta-analysts can make a substantial contribution to the literature and may overcome the aversion of clinicians for statistical reports, if they concentrate on the qualitative aspects of the analysis and "use statistics to clarify, not to obfuscate."[11(p246)]

References

1. Jenicek M. Meta-analysis in medicine: Where we are and where we want to go. J Clin Epidemiol 1989;42:35-44.
2. L'Abbe KA, Detsky AS, O'Rourke K. Meta-analysis in clinical research. Ann Intern Med 1987;107:224-33.
3. Glass GV, McGraw B, Smith ML. Meta-analysis in social research. Beverly Hills, CA: Sage Publications, 1981.
4. Light RJ, Pillemer DB. Summing up: The science of reviewing research. Cambridge, MA: Harvard University Press, 1984.
5. Hedges LV, Olkin I. Statistical methods for meta-analysis. Orlando, FL: Academic Press, 1985.
6. Cooper H, Hedges LV, eds. The handbook of research synthesis. New York: Russell Sage Foundation, 1994.
7. Moher D, Olkin I. Meta-analysis of randomized controlled trials: A concern for standards. JAMA 1995;274:1962-4.
8. Andersen JW. Meta-analyses need new publication standards (editorial). J Clin Oncol 1992;10:878-80.

9. Sacks HS, Berrier J, Reitman D, et al. Meta-analyses of randomized controlled trials. N Engl J Med 1987;316: 450-5.
10. Yusuf S, Simon R, Ellenberg S, eds. Methodologic issues in overviews of randomized clinical trials. Proceedings of a workshop sponsored by the National Heart, Lung, and Blood Institute and the National Cancer Institute. Stat Med 1987;6:217-409.
11. Goodman SN. Have you ever meta-analysis you didn't like? Ann Intern Med 1991;114:244-6.
12. Passamani E. Clinical trials: Are they ethical? N Engl J Med 1991;324:1589-91.
13. Hellman S, Hellman DS. Of mice but not men. Problems of the randomized clinical trial. N Engl J Med 1991;324: 1585-9. [Comment in N Engl J Med 1991;325:1513-9.]
14. Hennekens CH, Buring JE. Epidemiology in medicine. Boston, MA: Little Brown, 1987:30-53.
15. Chalmers TC, Levin H, Sacks HS, et al. Meta-analysis of clinical trials as a scientific discipline. I. Control of bias and comparison with large co-operative trials. Stat Med 1987;6:315-25.
16. Peto R. Why do we need systematic overviews of randomized trials? Stat Med 1987;6:233-40.
17. Yusuf S. Obtaining medically meaningful answers from an overview of randomized clinical trials. Stat Med 1987; 6:281-6.
18. Fleiss JL, Gross AJ. Meta-analysis in epidemiology, with special reference to studies of the association between exposure to environmental tobacco smoke and lung cancer: A critique. J Clin Epidemiol 1991;44:127-39.
19. Eysenck HJ. An exercise in megasilliness. Am Psychol 1978;35:517.
20. Wachter KW. Disturbed by meta-analysis? Science 1988; 241:1407-8.
21. O'Rourke K, Detsky AS. Meta-analysis in medical research: Strong encouragement for higher quality in individual research efforts. J Clin Epidemiol 1989;42:1021-4.
22. Mantel N, Haenszel W. Statistical aspects of the analysis of data from retrospective studies of disease. J Natl Cancer Inst 1959;22:719-48.
23. Yusuf S, Peto R, Lewis J, et al. Beta blockade during and after myocardial infarction: An overview of the randomized trials. Prog Cardiovasc Dis 1985;27:335-71.

24. Bordin JO, Heddle NM, Blajchman MA. Biologic effects of leukocytes present in transfused cellular blood products. Blood 1994;84:1703-21.
25. Blumberg N, Heal JM. Immunomodulation by blood transfusion: An evolving scientific and clinical challenge. Am J Med 1996;101:299-308.
26. Vamvakas EC, Blajchman MA. A proposal for an individual patient data-based meta-analysis of randomized controlled trials of allogeneic transfusion and postoperative bacterial infection. Transfus Med Rev 1997;11:180-94.
27. Duffy G, Neal KR. Differences in postoperative infection rates between patients receiving autologous and allogeneic blood transfusion: A meta-analysis of published randomized and nonrandomized studies. Transfus Med 1996;6:325-8.
28. Vamvakas E. Transfusion-associated cancer recurrence and infection: Meta-analysis of randomized, controlled clinical trials. Transfusion 1996;36:175-86.
29. Jensen LS, Andersen AJ, Christiansen PM, et al. Postoperative infection and natural killer cell function following blood transfusion in patients undergoing elective colorectal surgery. Br J Surg 1992;79:513-6.
30. Busch ORC, Hop WCJ, Hoynek van Papendrecht MAW, et al. Blood transfusion and prognosis in colorectal cancer. N Engl J Med 1993;328:1372-6.
31. Busch ORC, Hop WCJ, Marquet RL, et al. Autologous blood and infection after colorectal surgery (letter). Lancet 1994;343:668-9.
32. Heiss MM, Mempel W, Jauch KW, et al. Beneficial effect of autologous blood transfusion on infectious complications after colorectal cancer surgery. Lancet 1993;342:1328-33.
33. Houbiers JGA, Brand A, van de Watering LMG, et al. Randomized controlled trial comparing transfusion of leukocyte-depleted or buffy-coat-depleted blood in surgery for colorectal cancer. Lancet 1994;344:573-8.
34. Jensen LS, Kissmeyer-Nielsen P, Wolff B, et al. Randomized comparison of leukocyte-depleted versus buffy-coat-poor blood transfusion and complications after colorectal surgery. Lancet 1996;348:841-5.

35. Vamvakas EC, Carven JH, Hibberd PL. Blood transfusion and infection after colorectal cancer surgery. Transfusion 1996;36:1000-8.
36. Huque MF. Experiences with meta-analysis in FDA submissions. Proc Biopharmaceutical Section Am Stat Assoc 1988;2:28-33.
37. Dubey S. Regulatory considerations on meta-analysis and multicenter trials. Proc Biopharmaceutical Section Am Stat Assoc 1988;2:18-27.
38. Stein RA. Meta-analysis from one FDA reviewer's perspective. Proc Biopharmaceutical Section Am Stat Assoc 1988;2:34-8.
39. Elwood P. Causal relationships in medicine. New York: Oxford University Press, 1988.
40. Susser M. Judgment and causal inference: Critical in epidemiological studies. In: Susser M, ed, Epidemiology, health, and society: Selected papers. New York: Oxford University Press, 1988:69-81.
41. Sackett DL. Bias in analytic research. J Chron Dis 1979;32:51-63.
42. Vamvakas EC, Carven JH. Allogeneic blood transfusion, hospital charges, and length of hospitalization: A study of 487 consecutive patients undergoing colorectal cancer resection. Arch Pathol Lab Med 1998;122:145-51.
43. Vamvakas EC, Carven JH. Transfusion of white-cell-containing allogeneic blood components and postoperative wound infection: Effect of confounding factors. Transfus Med 1998;8:29-36.
44. Meares EM, Jr. Current patterns in nosocomial urinary tract infections. Urology 1991;37(Suppl 3):9-12.
45. Schlesselman JJ. Case-control studies: Design, conduct, analysis. New York: Oxford University Press, 1982:227-90.
46. Datta M. You cannot exclude the explanation you have not considered (facts, figures and fallacies). Lancet 1993;342:345-7.
47. Friedman LM, Furberg CD, DeMets DL. Fundamentals of clinical trials, 3rd ed. St Louis, MO: Mosby, 1995.
48. Green SB, Bryar DP. Using observational data from registries to compare treatments: The fallacy of omnimetrics. Stat Med 1984;3:361-70.

49. Wooley AL, Hogikyan ND, Geates GA, et al. Effect of blood transfusion on recurrence of head and neck carcinoma. Retrospective review and meta-analysis. Ann Otol Rhinol Laryngol 1992;101:724-30.
50. Chung M, Steinmetz OK, Gordon PH. Perioperative blood transfusion and outcome after resection for colorectal carcinoma. Br J Surg 1993;80:427-32.
51. Amato A, Pescatori M. Perioperative blood transfusion and outcome after resection for colorectal carcinoma. Br J Surg 1994;81:313-4.
52. Vamvakas E. Perioperative blood transfusion and cancer recurrence: Meta-analysis for explanation. Transfusion 1995;35:760-8.
53. Chalmers TC, Matta RJ, Smith H Jr, Kunzler AM. Evidence favoring the use of anticoagulants in the hospital phase of acute myocardial infarction. N Engl J Med 1977;297:1091-6.
54. Colditz GA, Miller JN, Mosteller F. How study design affects outcomes in comparisons of therapy, I: Medical. Stat Med 1989;8:441-54.
55. Miller JN, Colditz GA, Mosteller F. How study design affects outcomes in comparisons of therapy, II: Surgical. Stat Med 1989;8:455-66.
56. Easterbrook PJ, Berlin JA, Copalan R, Matthews DR. Publication bias in clinical research. Lancet 1991;337:867-72.
57. Relman AS. What a good medical journal does. The New York Times (Section IV) March 19, 1978:22.
58. Glantz SA. Biostatistics: How to detect, correct and prevent errors in the medical literature. Circulation 1980;61:1-7.
59. Evans M, Pollock AV. Trials on trial. A review of trials of antibiotic prophylaxis. Arch Surg 1984;119:109-13.
60. Pocock SJ, Hughes MD, Lee RJ. Statistical problems in the reporting of clinical trials. A survey of three medical journals. N Engl J Med 1987;317:426-32.
61. Altman DG. Statistics in medical journals. Stat Med 1982;1:59-71.
62. Gotzsche PC. Methodology and overt and hidden bias in reports of 196 double-blind trials of non-steroidal anti-inflammatory drugs in rheumatoid arthritis. Control Clin Trial 1989;10:31-56.

63. Pocock SJ, Lagakos SW. Practical experience of randomization in cancer trials: An international survey. Br J Cancer 1982;46:368-75.
64. Chalmers TC, Celano P, Sacks HS, et al. Bias in treatment assignment in controlled clinical trials. N Engl J Med 1983;309: 1358-61.
65. Lachin JM. Statistical properties of randomization in clinical trials. Control Clin Trial 1988;9:289-311.
66. Peto R. Why do we need systematic overviews of randomized trials? Stat Med 1987;6:233-44.
67. Chalmers TC, Smith H Jr, Blackburn B, et al. A method for assessing the quality of a randomized controlled trial. Control Clin Trial 1981;2:31-49.
68. Detsky AS, Naylor CD, O'Rourke K, et al. Incorporating variations in the quality of individual randomized trials into meta-analysis. J Clin Epidemiol 1992;45:255-65.
69. Zelen M. Guidelines for publishing papers on cancer clinical trials: Responsibilities of editors and authors. J Clin Oncol 1983;1:164-9.
70. Lichtenstein MJ, Mulrow CD, Elwood PC. Guidelines for reading case-control studies. J Chron Dis 1987;40:893-903.
71. Feinstein AR. Clinical epidemiology: The architecture of clinical research. Philadelphia, PA: Saunders, 1985: 543-7.
72. Liberati A, Himel HN, Chalmers TC. A quality assessment of randomized controlled trials of primary treatment of breast cancer. J Clin Oncol 1986;4:942-51.
73. International Committee of Medical Journal Editors. Uniform requirements for manuscript submitted to biomedical journals. Ann Intern Med 1988;108:258-65.
74. Simon R, Wittes RE. Methodologic guidelines for reports of clinical trials. Cancer Treat Rep 1985;69:1-3.
75. Begg C, Cho M, Eastwood S, et al. Improving the quality of reporting of randomized controlled trials. JAMA 1996; 276:637-9.
76. Rennie D. How to report randomized controlled trials: The Consort statement (editorial). JAMA 1996;276:649.
77. Peto R, Pike MC, Armitage P, et al. Design and analysis of randomized clinical trials requiring prolonged observation of each patient. I. Introduction and design. Br J Cancer 1976;34:585-612.

78. May GS, DeMets DL, Friedman LM, et al. The randomized clinical trial: Bias in the analysis. Circulation 1981; 64:669-73.
79. Collins R, Gray R, Godwin J, Peto R. Avoidance of large biases and large random errors in the assessment of moderate treatment effects: The need for systematic overviews. Stat Med 1987;6:245-50.
80. Halperin M, DeMets DL, Ware JH. Early methodological developments for clinical trials at the National Heart, Lung, and Blood Institute. Stat Med 1990;9:881-92.
81. Schultz KF, Chalmers I, Hayes RJ, Altman DG. Empirical evidence of bias: Dimensions of methodological quality associated with estimates of treatment effects in controlled trials. JAMA 1995;273:408-12.
82. Vamvakas EC. Meta-analysis in transfusion medicine. Transfusion 1997;37:329-45.
83. Gotzsche PC. Enalapril, atenolol, and hydrochlorothiazide in hypertension (letter). Lancet 1986;ii:38-9.
84. Karlowski TR, Chalmers TC, Frenkel LD, et al. Ascorbic acid for the common cold: A prophylactic and therapeutic trial. JAMA 1975;231:1038-42.
85. Huskisson EC, Scott J. How blind is double blind? And does it matter? Br J Clin Pharmacol 1976;3:331-2.
86. Sackett DL, Gent M. Controversy in counting and attributing events in clinical trials. N Engl J Med 1979;301:1410-2.
87. Steinberg KK, Thacker SB, Smith SJ, et al. A meta-analysis of the effect of estrogen replacement therapy on the risk of breast cancer. JAMA 1991;265:1985-90.
88. Klein S, Simes J, Blackburn GL. Total parenteral nutrition and cancer clinical trials. Cancer 1986;58:1378-86.
89. Berlin JA, Colditz GA. A meta-analysis of physical activity in the prevention of coronary heart disease. Am J Epidemiol 1990;142:612-28.
90. Laird NM, Mosteller F. Some statistical methods for combining experimental results. Int J Tech Assess Health Care 1990;6:5-30.
91. Borzak S, Ridker PM. Discordance between meta-analyses and large-scale randomized controlled trials: Examples from the management of acute myocardial infarction. Ann Intern Med 1995;123:873-7.

92. Bailar JC III. The promise and problems of meta-analysis (editorial). N Engl J Med 1997;337:559-61.
93. Meta-analysis under scrutiny (editorial). Lancet 1997; 350:675.
94. Villar J, Carroli G, Belizan JM. Predictive ability of meta-analyses of randomized controlled trials. Lancet 1995; 345:772-6.
95. Cappelleri JC, Ioannidis JPA, Schmid CH, et al. Large trials vs meta-analyses of small trials: How do their results compare? JAMA 1996;276:1332-8.
96. LeLorier J, Gregoire B, Benhaddad A, et al. Discrepancies between meta-analyses and subsequent large randomized, controlled trials. N Engl J Med 1997;337:536-42.
97. Ioannidis JPA, Cappelleri JC, Lau J. Issues in comparisons between meta-analyses and large trials. JAMA 1998; 279:1089-93.

In: Brecher ME, Busch MP, eds.
Research Design and Analysis
Bethesda, MD: American Association of Blood Banks, 1998

3

Statistical Analysis

Michael H. Kanter, MD

BIOLOGIC SYSTEMS ARE INCREDIBLY complex systems. Thus, where many laws of physical sciences can be described by mathematical equations, most major breakthroughs in biologic science have historically originated from qualitative observations.[1,2] More recently, biological systems have been described by mathematical equations (models). One advantage of a mathematical model is that the language of mathematics is more precise than qualitative reasoning. As a result, ambiguities should be nonexistent or infrequent at most. If all assumptions and terms are clearly understood, a mathematical model can be a very powerful tool. If, on the other hand, an assumption is violated or a term misunderstood, serious errors may result.

Several examples of mathematical models have been used in transfusion medicine. Models of preoperative autologous donation,[3] transfusion-associated graft-vs-host disease,[4] and window period transfusion-transmitted disease incidences[5,6] are some examples. Unlike qualitative experiments, once a series of assumptions is stated and mathematical terms defined, anyone can use the model and theoretically arrive at the same conclusions. Thus, when a mathematical model is derived, all of the assumptions should be clearly

Michael H. Kanter, MD, Director of Transfusion Medicine, Southern California Permanente Medical Group, Department of Pathology, Kaiser Permanente, Woodland Hills, California, and Associate Clinical Professor of Pathology, University of California, Los Angeles, California

stated and justified in any report. Without these assumptions, the reader cannot critically analyze the article and, more important, may not be able to properly apply the knowledge in the article to future patients or situations.

Statistical Analysis as a Type of Mathematical Model

Statistical analysis is often viewed as a highly abstract mystical method of calculating results that is beyond the grasp of biomedical researchers. If, however, one views statistical analysis merely as a type of mathematical model, some of the mystery of statistics may become more clear. One merely has to develop a set of assumptions, define some terms, and use the very precise language of mathematics to describe the system one is analyzing. Just as with all mathematical models, all of the assumptions made in the analysis should be clear to the researcher and reader. If not, there is the potential for misinterpretation. Once all of the assumptions are stated or known and agreed upon, there should be general agreement on the conclusions. Although statistical analysis deals with random variation while many mathematical models are completely deterministic, the basic process of constructing a mathematical description of a system is similar.

It is unfortunate that statistical analysis is sometimes relegated to a subordinate role in experimental design and analysis. Unlike the mathematical models noted above, the assumptions used in the statistical analysis are either not stated or are ignored. Disregard for these assumptions may lead to erroneous conclusions or inappropriate application of the data. More important, the meaning of many terms and quantities that have very precise definitions are often misunderstood or used in an imprecise fashion. Space limitations do not allow an article in a biomedical journal to repeat the definition of such commonly used terms as a p value or a standard deviation. Both the authors and readers are assumed to be familiar with the assumptions behind common statistical terms and tests.

A previous article by this author delineated many statistical errors that occur in transfusion medicine literature.[7] It was noted that these errors are common in many prestigious medical journals in many specialties. An accompanying editorial[8] correctly noted that the statistical errors that were delineated in that article had a rather narrow focus. This editorial noted that there are many statistical practices that are not obviously erroneous, yet still may lead to much confusion and misinterpretation.

This chapter addresses some of the concerns raised in that editorial by discussing some of the major assumptions made in statistical analysis. Examples of such assumptions in the transfusion medicine literature are given. Precise definitions of some statistical terms are provided, emphasizing those practices that might be technically correct but still may lead to confusion or differences in interpretation. In particular, the meaning of the p value and the assumptions behind hypothesis testing are explained.

The Importance of p Values in Medical Research

Medical researchers are often under pressure to publish their findings. One important determinant of how likely a study is to be published is whether or not a manuscript based on the study contains a p value <0.05. Easterbrook et al[9] noted that studies with statistically significant results were more likely to be published than those finding no difference between the study groups (odds ratio 2.32). This publication bias was largely attributed to failure of the investigator to submit the study for publication. Similar findings were also noted by Dickersin et al.[10]

A bias toward publication of positive studies has the potential to interfere with the conclusions of meta-analysis or qualitative reviews of the literature. Just as important, however, is that investigators, armed with knowledge of this publication bias, may attempt to "find" statistically significant results by using multiple comparisons, post hoc comparisons not anticipated before data collection (see below), or a variety of other clever devices. The p value is often equated with success. If an investigator reports a p value greater than the magical 0.05, he or she is not infrequently said to have "failed" to find statistical significance. Viewing this as a "failure" is assuming that statistically significant results should have been obtained in the first place and that somehow the investigators did something wrong. Given our current overemphasis on obtaining p values less than 0.05, it should not be suprising that investigators are reluctant to publish "negative" findings. Much of this overemphasis can be corrected by better understanding what a p value really is.

The Meaning of the p Value

A p value is a conditional probability. It is the probability that one would obtain the result observed or more extreme results *given that the null hypothesis is true.*[11,12] The null hypothesis is a fact postulated to be true prior to the data collection. Usually it states that two or more groups are equal with respect to some variable. Sometimes it may state that one variable has no relationship to one or more other variables. The p value does not indicate the probability that the null hypothesis is true. In calculating a p value, one first assumes that the null hypothesis is true. The p value is then the probability of obtaining the data one has collected or obtaining data that deviates even more from the null hypothesis.

If the p value is <0.05, a result is deemed to be statistically significant, and if it is >0.05, it is deemed to be not statistically significant. Thus, the p value is used to dichotomize the results into "significant" or "not significant." Before examining the interpretation of the p value in detail, however, it is important to understand many of the assumptions made in statistical testing.

Assumptions Made in Statistical Testing

Each statistical test has its own unique set of assumptions; however, there are many assumptions that are common to most of the more frequently performed tests. These assumptions are usually not explicitly stated, presumably because they are considered too obvious. Unfortunately, the obvious is sometimes forgotten. These assumptions are listed in Table 3-1.

Absence of Confounding Variables

In measuring the difference in value of a variable between two or more groups, a researcher typically assumes that there are

Table 3-1. Assumptions of Most Statistical Tests

* No confounding variables are present.
* If randomization was performed, it was done correctly.
* Results can be applied to other patient populations (generalizability).
* Measurements made repeatedly on the same subject are not the same as measurements made on different subjects.
* Statistical tests are specified before examination of data.
* Starting and stopping times of data collection are independent of results.
* All statistical tests performed are published.

no confounding variables. A confounding variable is one that is associated with the variable of interest and is distributed differently in the two groups.[13] Any statistically significant difference in the value of the variable of interest between the groups may then be due partially or entirely to the confounding variable. Thus, if one finds a statistically significantly higher hemoglobin in patients with disease A (90% of whom are men) vs patients with disease B (90% of whom are women), one cannot conclude that disease B is associated with a lower hemoglobin. The difference might be explained by the confounding variable (gender), which is associated with the difference in hemoglobin.

It cannot be overemphasized that the confounding variable may or may not be known. Disregard for confounding variables is common in studies on the safety of directed as compared with allogeneic donors, where the percentage of first-time donors (a confounding variable) is ignored.[14]

Confounding variables might also have affected some studies on the utility of transfusion audits.[15] In some of these transfusion audit studies, transfusion audits were initiated near the same time as awareness of acquired immune deficiency syndrome (AIDS) became widespread, resulting in a marked change toward a more conservative transfusion practice. Therefore, any statistically significant decrease in transfusion rates might have been due at least in part to the change in transfusion practice created by fear of AIDS, rather than by any transfusion audits. Concomitant use of informed consent[16] and introduction of multiple other interventions at the time of the initiation of the transfusion audit also have been suggested to be potentially confounding variables.[15,16]

It has also been suggested that nonrandomized studies concerning whether transfusion increases the risk of cancer recurrence are biased because of many (known and unknown) confounding variables that are associated with both transfusion and a higher risk of recurrence.[17] The solution to the problem of confounding variables is either to perform randomized controlled studies, which should eliminate the effect of any confounding variables, or to perform more sophisticated multivariate analysis, which can statistically adjust for any known confounding variables.

If Randomization Was Performed, It Was Done Correctly

As noted above, confounding variables may lead to spurious conclusions. In order to prevent this, investigators use randomization. The hope is to ensure that any confounding variables are distributed similarly in the groups being studied.

Of concern is the fact that 5-10% of "randomized" trials have been noted to use nonrandom methods of allocation.[18,19] Methods such as alternation (using odd and even birth dates or hospital numbers) are not truly random and may allow physicians to know in advance the group to which a patient will be assigned. Accordingly, these practices may allow physician bias in the assignment of patients into the treatment groups.[19] Altman and Dore[20] noted that only 49% of trials specified how random numbers were generated (eg, random number tables, computer, etc). Knowing that not all randomized trials are truly randomized, one is left with some doubt about whether randomization truly occurred, unless the method of randomization was stated.

There are several types of randomization.[11] In simple randomization, the investigator uses a random method to assign patients to different groups. If done properly, there should be approximately equal numbers of patients in each group. One would expect, however, that random variation will cause some slight unevenness in group size. Blocked randomization allows the investigator to randomly assign patients in multiple small increments so that the final numbers of patients in each group are more likely to be equal. In two disturbing reviews of randomized studies, the sample sizes of the two groups tended to be more similar than would be expected by chance.[20,21] Although the findings of these reviews could have been due to unreported blocking, the authors speculated that it is possible that investigators may have either used a nonrandom system such as alternation or added extra patients to one group when an imbalance was noted.

Results Can Be Applied to Other Patient Populations (Generalizability)

Generalizability is the applicability of a study to other types of situations. The implications of the issue of generalizability may best be understood through example. An investigator makes an observation of one or more groups of patients; for example, the hemoglobin level before and after preoperative autologous donation. If one were interested only in that particular set of patients, there would be no reason to perform any statistical tests. Any decrease in hemoglobin would be exactly that observed in the particular set of patients.

Most of the time, however, one is interested in applying the measured decrease in hemoglobin to other sets of patients. These may be patients to be seen at the same institution in the future or patients seen at other institutions. In the autologous donation example, any decrease in hemoglobin in the measured patients may be slightly different from that found in a new set of patients. Statistical methods may be used for measurement of this expected variation in the decrease in hemoglobin. This is usually done by calculating a standard deviation, a 95% confidence interval, or some percentiles. If one were interested in whether or not the hemoglobin decreased, one would calculate a p value. The results of these statistical analyses are then generalized and presumed to apply to other patient populations.

The investigator in this autologous donation example may publish the findings of a decrease in hemoglobin resulting from autologous donation. However, problems may arise if the measured decrease is extrapolated to other populations of patients who are somehow different. Often it is not the original investigator who encounters these problems. For example, Kasper et al[22] reported a minimal decrease in hemoglobin resulting from preoperative autologous donations.

However, in that study, all of the autologous donors were required to have a hematocrit of 36% or greater. If one were to try to extrapolate these results to a different population of autologous donors in which the minimum acceptable hematocrit is 33%, one might be severely disappointed. For example, several investigators who have allowed hematocrits as low as 33% have found much larger decreases in hemoglobin of up to 1 mg/dL per unit donated.[23-26] Differences in the decrease in hemoglobin may also be due to a variety of factors other than the difference in hematocrit, including interval between donations and surgery, size of the patients, iron stores of the patients, general health of the patients, etc. It is the duty of the investigator to clearly define as many of the relevant characteristics of the study subjects as possible. It is also the duty of the reader to be careful in applying results of a study to a population that might differ from the study population in one or more important factors. The above example dealt with descriptive statistics; however, the assumption that results can be generalized to other populations applies to statistical hypothesis testing as well.

Studies of the utility of transfusion audits may be another area in which statistically significant results may not be generalizable.[15] Many studies that report decreases in blood use due to transfusion audits are from institutions with a high underlying rate of inappropriate transfusion. These high rates of inappropriate transfusion contrast with a recent national survey that found that the inappropriate red cell transfusion rates detected by hospital transfusion monitoring systems averaged less than 1%.[27] Any decreases in red cell use reported by institutions with a high rate of inappropriate red cell transfusion may not be applicable to institutions with much lower rates of inappropriate use. (It is not relevant for this discussion whether or not the institutions reporting such low rates of inappropriate use truly have such low rates or whether they are merely not identifying the inappropriate transfusions.)

Another example of generalizability of results is the study of Bowden et al[28] (see below) that purported to demonstrate equivalence of cytomegalovirus (CMV)-seronegative blood and filtered blood. Wenz[29] noted that Bowden et al[28] used only one type of leukocyte-reduction filter in their study and has argued that the results may not be generalizable to the use of other filters.

It should be emphasized that the generalizability of a study is a different issue from the validity of a study. A study may have been performed and interpreted correctly but may not be applicable in all situations. It may be that the reader of a study is the one who commits the mistake of ignoring the issue of generalizability rather than the author of the study. Moreover, arguments over whether a study is generalizable are often based on speculation or hunches. Thus, Wenz[29] may or may not be correct in his concern about generalizing the results of the study of Bowden et al[28] to other types of filtration.

Measurements Made Repeatedly on the Same Subject Are Not the Same as Measurements Made on Different Subjects

Suppose that one studies the incidence of infectious disease markers in autologous donors and allogeneic donors. Assume that one compares the prevalence of an infectious disease marker over time and finds that there are 8/192 (4.2%) positive autologous donors vs 16/784 (2.0%) positive allogeneic donors (p = 0.16). If, on the other hand, all autologous donors gave 4 units (the donors with a positive test are not deferred and all test results remain unchanged), then there would be 32/768 (4.2%) positive autologous units vs 16/784 (2%) allogeneic units (p = 0.03). Thus, on the same data, analyzing donors yields a nonstatistically significant result, while analyzing donations yields a statistically significant result. The reason for this is that in analyzing donations, one is making a repeated measurement on the same donor and analyzing these measurements as if they were made on different donors. It should be noted that nonstatistical arguments have been put forth on the advantages and disadvantages of measuring donors vs donations.[30,31] Discussion of these arguments is beyond the scope of this chapter.

In the usual case, measurements are made repeatedly on the same subject when it is difficult to enroll enough patients in a study. This author has seen several studies of the response to platelet transfusions in which multiple transfusions are given to a series of consecutively treated patients and the results are analyzed as if each transfusion had been given to a different patient. When data are incorrectly analyzed in this way, it gives the investigator a greater sample size. As noted by Bland and Altman,[32] most statistics texts do not warn against ignoring the fact that data may have been collected on the same individuals more than once. They further note that "It is so ingrained in statisticians that this is a bad idea that it never occurs to them that anyone would do it." If one is forced to make repeated measurements on the same patients, one should consult a knowledgeable statistician.

Statistical Tests Are Specified Before Examination of Data

It seems somewhat obvious that the statistical test to be performed should be specified before collection of the data. Each statistical test has a 5% chance of finding statistical significance when none exists. If an investigator performs enough analysis, he or she will find some statistically significant results when none exists. When one does not specify ahead of time what comparisons will be subject to statistical analysis, there is a tendency to examine the data and choose to perform statistical tests on only those results that appear to be statistically significant. This practice will tend to increase the rate of falsely finding statistical significance when none exists. Unfortunately, it is tempting to look through data after collection, find results that may appear statistically significant, and then decide to perform a statistical test to prove that indeed there is statistical significance. Much of this temptation arises from the fact that obtaining a statistically significant p value is associated with a greater chance of publication (see above). This type of post hoc statistical testing of results often is referred to as data dredging or fishing and is well known to statisticians.[11]

The most commonly used example of this error in blood banking is the use of p values in antibody identification.[33] In this situation, one performs an antibody panel, examines the results to see which of many different antibody patterns fits best, and then relies on a rule of thumb as to how many antigen-positive cells must react and how many antigen-negative cells must not react. This rule of thumb is based on a p value that assumes that the blood banker specified which antibody is present prior to examination of the panel. Unlike antibody identification, however, one cannot know if the authors of a research article are guilty of data dredging unless they admit to it.

Starting and Stopping Times of Data Collection Are Independent of the Results

Blood bankers are often interested in the frequency of certain occurrences (eg, rates of bacterial contamination of units, transfusion-transmitted-disease marker rates, or transfusion reaction rates). In measuring such rates, one should not choose the starting and stopping time of the data collection after starting to collect data. This is analogous to data dredging. Suppose, for example, that an investigator notices that a few units of platelets are contaminated with bacteria in June. Curiosity aroused, the investigator then starts measuring the percentage of contaminated units for the months of June and July. It would be erroneous to extrapolate that rate to other institutions or to other periods in the same institution because the results are upwardly biased; the period of data collection included a time already known to be associated with contaminated units.

For example, Yomtovian et al[34] noted two patients who received bacterially contaminated platelet transfusions. In order to eliminate the upward bias, they correctly performed a *prospective* study. The contamination rate of their platelets was 0.19% and did not *retrospectively* include the first two cases they noted. An earlier report,[35] however, had been published that included the first two retrospective cases and reported a higher rate of contamination (0.4%). This earlier report (not unjustifiably) was published presumably in order to alert blood bankers to the problem of bacterial contamination in a more timely fashion rather than wait for prospective data to be collected.

This problem of bias in measuring rates occurs mainly when a study is retrospective and the rates being observed are quite small. Although the example given above dealt with simple measurement of a crude rate, the same problem arises with performance of statistical tests to compare rates in different groups. Although a definite stopping time may not be set ahead of time when one has planned one or more interim analyses, this type of analysis requires special statistical methods (see section on sequential statistical testing). A retrospective study must provide enough information to ensure the readers that the starting and stopping times of the study were not influenced by the events being measured. Unlike the well-described prospective report of Yomtovian et al,[34] not all retrospective studies provide this information.

All Statistical Tests Performed Are Published

In previous paragraphs, the issue of publication bias was noted. Lack of awareness of this issue can cause an incorrect perception of the results of published studies. Specifically, a reader of the medical literature will be examining a biased collection of research. Even though the p values in each article may be correct, reading a biased sample of positive studies may lead one to incorrectly believe that a positive relationship exists. This problem with publication bias is not confined to meta-analysis. This problem of publication bias has been postulated to be more severe in smaller studies.[36,37]

As an example, suppose that it is of interest to determine if there is a difference in hemoglobin between Rh-positive and Rh-negative individuals. An experiment is planned in which the researchers measure and compare (using a t test) the hemoglobin levels of 10 Rh-negative and 10 Rh-positive individuals. Suppose that this experiment is performed in 40 laboratories or done 40 times in one laboratory. With a p value of 0.05 or less to indicate significance, even though there is no difference in hemoglobin levels between the two groups, one would expect two experiments to find a statistically significant difference and 38 experiments to find no statistically significant difference. If the results of the 38 "negative experiments" are not published, a reader of the medical literature will see only the two positive studies and be tempted to conclude that there is a difference in hemoglobin between Rh-positive and Rh-negative individuals.

Use of Too Many p Values

Given the emphasis placed on obtaining statistically significant p values, it should not be surprising that researchers frequently perform analyses that generate too many p values.[7] There are several ways in which too many p values may be generated. Each arises in a slightly different situation; however, all share the problem of increasing the likelihood of obtaining statistical significance when none exists. As noted previously, each time a p value is calculated, there is a chance that it is falsely statistically significant. Four ways in which one might generate a false statistical significance are outlined in Table 3-2 and discussed below.

Use of Too Many Variables for Comparison

One way to increase the likelihood of a falsely significant p value is for the investigator to compare two groups using multiple variables. For example, several studies have been performed to determine the relative safety of autologous units or directed donor units as compared with allogeneic units. A researcher in this area typically measures rates of positivity for seven infectious disease tests.[1] If one of these rates of positivity is higher at the 0.05 level of significance in the autologous or directed donor group than in the allogeneic group, investigators may interpret this to indicate that autologous or directed units are less safe. However, one is measuring seven different rates that are approximately independent.[14] If the two groups were identical with respect to all rates, one would still have a 5% chance of falsely finding a statistically significant difference for each marker measured. The probability of falsely finding one or more differences is approximately $7 \times 0.05 = 0.35$. The simplest way of correcting for this is to use a level of significance of $0.05/7 = 0.008$ (Bonferroni method).[11] This correction is sometimes,[38] but not always, performed. Multivariate analysis may also circumvent the problem of multiple variables.

Table 3-2. Various Ways in Which Too Many p Values Can Be Generated

* Use of too many variables for comparison.
* Multiple pairwise comparisons among many groups.
* Subgroup analysis.
* Sequential statistical testing.

Another common type of study in blood banking in which multiple comparisons may be made is when an investigator attempts to find an association between a disease and HLA types. The number of alleles of the HLA system allows the investigator to calculate a p value for each of the many different alleles. The Bonferroni method would alleviate the problem of falsely finding a significant result, which would otherwise be generated by the use of multiple p values.

Multiple Pairwise Comparisons Among Many Groups

Comparing one variable among three or more groups is another way in which multiple p values arise. If there are n groups, then there are $n!/[2!(n-2)!]$ possible pairwise comparisons where the "!" sign indicates factorial. Thus, for four groups of patients there are six possible pairwise comparisons and six p values (eg, group 1 vs 2, 1 vs 3, 1 vs 4, 2 vs 3, 2 vs 4, and 3 vs 4). Each p value has a 5% chance of being falsely positive when there is no actual difference between groups. This problem has been noted before in the transfusion medicine literature[7] and can be corrected by using analysis of variance or specialized multiple comparison methods.[39] If, instead, multiple pairwise comparisons are performed and published, the reader can correct for this by multiplying the p value (assuming it is given instead of the often-used p<0.05) by the number of pairwise comparisons.[39]

Subgroup Analysis

Multiple p values arise when multiple subgroups of patients in a study are analyzed. Usually, a study is performed and a p value is calculated for the main results. These global results, however, may not be helpful in developing a treatment plan for individual patients. The authors then analyze their data to determine if there are any interesting trends in various subgroups of their patients or samples. They then attempt to calculate more p values based on these various subgroups of the data. If the authors do not specify ahead of time what their main analysis was and merely perform multiple separate statistical tests to calculate a variety of p values for various subgroups, they will likely find some that show statistical significance.[37,40] More sophisticated multivariate statistical tests are available that allow one to test for interactions among variables (subgroups); however, subgroup analysis should generally be interpreted cautiously.[37] Subgroup analysis should be specified prior to collection of data and should have some biologically plausible basis.[40] The p value for the primary analysis should be given the most weight and any so-called secondary or subgroup analysis should be viewed merely as an interesting speculation that needs further confirmation. Often, published articles do not state their primary analysis and, in fact, the authors may not have had one at the outset. In some cases, the investigators may no longer remember which hypotheses were truly postulated in advance and which were derived from the data, or which were a priori considered plausible and which were not.[40] This allows the authors to generate spurious statistically significant results more easily.

Sometimes, however, the goal of the article is to show that there is no difference between groups (eg, the goal is to find p >0.05). In this case, each time one performs a secondary or subgroup analysis, one runs the risk of finding a statistically significant result that would raise doubts about the demonstration of equivalency. This risk is exemplified in the Bowden et al study[28] of transfusion-transmitted CMV infection in patients undergoing marrow transplantation. In that study, the primary analysis was of CMV that occurred 21-100 days after transplantation. A secondary analysis was of CMV that occurred anytime after transplantation. The primary analysis showed no statistical difference; however, the secondary analysis did show a statistically significant difference. The secondary analysis was correctly given less weight by the authors. Opinions, however, may differ as to how much less weight one should give to secondary analyses. The answer is not a statistical one, but rather one of judgment and opinion.

Sequential Statistical Testing

Sometimes, an investigator may collect data over time. Ideally, the investigator should decide ahead of time when the experiment will be terminated and the data analyzed. Suppose, however, that the investigator examines the data at some point and finds that the p value is close to but greater than 0.05. The investigator then decides to collect more data and reexamine and test the data later, hoping to find statistical significance. This type of analysis, like those mentioned above, generates too many p values. The first time one performs the statistical test, there is a 0.05 probability of falsely concluding significance when none exists. On the second analysis, there is a second chance (with its associated probability) of falsely concluding significance when none exists. The total chance of falsely concluding significance is the sum of the two probabilities and therefore becomes greater than the 0.05 originally desired. Complex methods of sequential analysis that correct for this problem are available; generally, they involve the use of a lower p value at each step of less than 0.05.[41] If the investigator does not admit to the sequential testing (perhaps he or she is unaware of the potential problems affecting sequential testing), and only reports the statistically significant p value, the reader will be unable to detect this error. One area in which the problems inherent in sequential statistical testing are often ignored is antibody identification.[33] In this situation, one tests a serum against samples of red cells with known antigens. A p value is calculated on the basis of the number of positive and negative reactions. If the p value obtained for a given antibody identification approaches but is not less than 0.05, one tests more cells until the p value becomes less than 0.05. This p value is spuriously low because the impact of sequential testing is ignored.

What p Values Do Not Indicate

The definition of a p value was given previously. A complete understanding of this definition requires that one know what types of information p values do *not* provide. These types of information are discussed below and summarized in Table 3-3.

Statistically Insignificant p Values Do Not Indicate That There Is No Difference Between Two or More Groups

Usually, an investigator wants to find a difference between two or more groups based on a theoretical reason why they should be different. Sometimes, however, the goal of a study is to show that two groups are the same. For example, a re-

Table 3-3. What p Values Do Not Indicate

* The probability that a difference exists between two groups.
* The magnitude of a difference between two groups.
* Whether one treatment or process is better than another.
* Whether a true difference exists between two groups.
* Whether results are clinically significant.
* Whether there are differences in baseline variables in randomized groups.
* Whether two groups of results are equivalent.

searcher might want to show that a new, less expensive method is equivalent to the existing standard method. If a study results in a p value >0.05, this means that the investigator has not found a statistically significant difference between the two groups, but this does not necessarily allow one to conclude that there is no actual difference between the two groups. If one concludes on the basis of p>0.05 that no difference exists, one runs the risk of committing a so-called type II error.[42]

In order to understand how one may find no statistically significant difference between two groups that are indeed different, it is important to remember that the p value is a mathematical quantity that is affected not only by the difference between two groups, but also by the sample size and the variation in the population of the characteristic being measured. Suppose that treatment A is effective 50% of the time and treatment B is effective 49% of the time. Table 3-4 lists the outcomes (p values) for several different sample sizes in a hypothetical experiment comparing treatments A and B. For each sample size in Table 3-4, the difference between the two treatments is the same. Note that for the smaller sample sizes, the p value is quite large. As the sample size increases, the p value falls and eventually goes below 0.05. Thus, depending on the sample size, the p value may vary widely even if the difference is held constant.

Generally, the investigator must decide, in advance, how much "difference" between two groups can exist without being clinically important. The needed sample size of the study is then calculated based on this "difference," the expected

Table 3-4. Number of Survivors Using Treatments A and B for Various Sample Sizes, Assuming Equal Numbers of Patients in Each Treatment

Sample Size	Treatment A	Treatment B	p Value
100	50 (50%)	49 (49%)	0.99
1000	500 (50%)	490 (49%)	0.69
2000	1000 (50%)	980 (49%)	0.55
4000	2000 (50%)	1960 (49%)	0.38
8000	4000 (50%)	3920 (49%)	0.21
10000	5000 (50%)	4900 (49%)	0.16
12000	6000 (50%)	5800 (49%)	0.13
20000	10000 (50%)	9800 (49%)	0.046

variation in the sample population of the factor being measured, the level of significance required (usually 0.05), and the required probability of finding a difference when one exists (power).[11,36] If the allowable "difference" is not agreed upon, then there may be great differences in the interpretation of the study.

It should be noted that the maximal allowable difference that is considered clinically unimportant is a subjective medical decision and should not be left for the statistician to decide alone. In practice, the determination of the sample size may involve some negotiations. If the initial desired sample size is too large to be practical, the investigator may elect either to tolerate a larger difference, to increase the chance of a false-negative result (use a lower power), to increase the level of significance required, or to increase the sample size.[36] These determinations require judgment, and common sense is required. A survey of "negative" clinical trials found that type II errors were frequent, with many studies being unable to detect as much as a 50% difference in therapeutic success.[42]

As noted above, sometimes an investigator wants to demonstrate that the two treatments are equivalent. Thus, unlike most studies, the investigator desires p to be greater than 0.05. In many cases, a 1% difference in survival, as shown in Table 3-4, is not deemed clinically different and the choice between treatment A and treatment B is made based on other factors (eg, side effects, treatment-related morbidity, response time of treatment, cost, etc). The public, however, has been urging the blood banking community to provide a zero-risk blood supply, with patients and physicians often appearing to ignore costs or other factors.[43] This situation has the potential to make the design and interpretation of studies looking for equivalence extremely difficult.

In a very strict sense, equivalence can be defined as follows: Two sets M and N are said to be equivalent if there is a one-to-one correspondence between the elements of M and the elements of N.[44] In essence, two treatments are equivalent if each and every person responds exactly the same to one treatment as he or she does to the other. In practice, this is never the case and one must arbitrarily create a practical definition of equivalence.

The easiest way to deal with this problem of equivalence is to do away with hypothesis testing and p values. Instead, one calculates confidence intervals (CI) for the difference in treatments (see below).[45] If the upper limit of the confidence interval of the difference is less than a specified amount (d), then equivalence is demonstrated. Typically, one uses a one-sided CI because one is only interested in knowing whether the experimental treatment is equal to or better than the standard treatment.[46]

Alternatively, some statisticians have advocated a different fashion of determining equivalence using hypothesis testing.[47,48] Instead of using a null hypothesis of no difference, one can create a null hypothesis that there is a difference greater than or equal to a specified amount, and then attempt to disprove this hypothesis. For example, assume that the success rate is p^s and p^e for a standard vs an experimental treatment, respectively. Instead of using the usual null hypothesis H_0: $p^s = p^e$, one uses the null hypothesis H_0: $p^s > p^e + d$ where d is the largest difference allowable for the two treatments to be considered equivalent. The new null hypothesis is that the treatments are not equivalent. Now rejecting the null hypothesis and concluding equivalence involves the usual situation of finding p to be less than 0.05. The interested reader is referred to the original articles for details of the statistical calculations.[47,48] In general, the confidence interval method will yield equivalent results.

This problem of equivalency is illustrated in the prospective randomized trial by Bowden et al[28] comparing CMV-seronegative blood components to filtered blood components. The authors of this well-designed study stated that the projected incidence of CMV infection and/or disease was 1-3% and that any difference less than or equal to 5% was clinically insignificant. Based on these estimates, a sample size of 500 (250 in each arm) was deemed to be needed to be 80% certain of finding a statistically significant result.

One needs to decide if a "difference" this size is important in this context. The authors, in their primary analysis, found a nonstatistically significant "difference" of CMV disease (1.2% in the filtered group vs 0% in the seronegative group; p = 0.25). On the basis of this result, the authors concluded that filtered blood and CMV-seronegative blood are equivalent in terms of risk of CMV disease transmission. This position has been endorsed by the AABB[49] as well as by a recent review article.[50] Others,[51,52] however, disagreed on the basis that the rate of serious CMV disease in the study was greater in the filtered blood, irrespective of the statistically nonsignificant p value. The Food and Drug Administration[53] also disagreed with the conclusions of Bowden et al,[28] in part on the basis that the study demonstrated efficacy, but not to the point of equivalence.

The fundamental issue raised by this study is how different the measured rates can be and still be considered "equivalent." The answer to this question is not statistical but is rather a matter of judgment, depending on a balance of issues such as incidence and mortality from CMV-disease, cost of treating CMV disease, cost and availability of CMV-seronegative blood, reliability of bedside leukocyte-reduction filters in a noncontrolled study, etc. If one deems a difference of approximately 1% to be clinically important, the sample size of a study necessary to prove equivalence may be prohibitively large and unlikely to ever be achieved.

Suppose, on the other hand, that one deems a difference of approximately 1-5% to be clinically insignificant. Also suppose that a large enough study were done that demonstrated identical results as that of Bowden et al[28] (1.2% CMV disease in the leukocyte-reduction group vs 0% in the seronegative group) but was statistically significant (p<0.05) because of the larger sample size. The interpretation should still be that filtered and seronegative blood were equivalent in terms of CMV transmission despite the statistically significant p value.

There is no universally accepted definition of how close the results of two treatments must be in order to be considered equivalent. The definition in large part depends upon what is being studied and its context. In a recent study on tissue plasminogen activator for acute myocardial infarction,[54] equivalence between two different dosage schedules was defined as a difference of 0.44% or less. On the other hand, it has been suggested that a difference as high as 6% might be appropriate in equivalency studies for reducing perinatal transmission of the human immunodeficiency virus in developing countries.[55]

A well-conducted equivalency study should always state its criteria for equivalency, which must be set prior to the trial. Many times, however, investigators may not realize that they are performing an equivalency study. They may not set criteria for equivalency and, instead, automatically set the criteria at a p value of greater than 0.05. One type of equivalency study in transfusion medicine is a comparison of a conservative to a more liberal transfusion policy. It is improper to conclude equivalency in this area when investigators merely show no statistical difference between using two different transfusion "triggers."

Statistically Significant p Values Alone Do Not Indicate the Likelihood That a Difference Exists Between Two Groups

The "bottom line" in statistics is often indicated by a p value. When a statistically significant result (p<0.05) is generated, many investigators incorrectly interpret this to indicate that the likelihood that the correct conclusion was drawn is 95%. Although widely used and stated, this interpretation is incorrect. *The p value does not indicate how likely the investigators' conclusions are to be correct.* Clearly, understanding the meaning of a p value will prevent such misinterpretation.[56]

Before an investigator begins collecting data, he or she specifies a null hypothesis (H_0). The data are collected and analyzed to either prove or disprove the null hypothesis. If one assumes that the null hypothesis is correct, the p value is the probability of obtaining the study results or obtaining study results even more different from the null hypothesis than the study results. If one rejects the null hypothesis based on the study results, the p value is the probability of rejecting the null hypothesis given that it is true. Mathematically,

$$p = \text{prob}(\text{reject } H_0 / H_0 \text{ is true})$$
(Equation 1)

where the "/" sign indicates a conditional probability and is often read as "given." Thus, if one uses a p value of 0.05 to reject the null hypothesis and indicate statistical significance, it means that if one were to conduct the same experiment 100 times and the null hypothesis were true, one would falsely conclude that the null hypothesis is not true about five times.

What the investigator is really interested in, however, is a different conditional probability.[57,58] If he or she conducts a study and finds a statistically significant result, the investigator wants to know the probability that H_0 is false given that the experiment yielded statistically significant results. This can be denoted by

$$\text{prob}(H_0 \text{ is false} / \text{reject } H_0)$$
(Equation 2)

The p value is often incorrectly interpreted as $p = (H_0$ is true/reject $H_0)$ instead of the probability in equation 1. All is not lost, however, even though one is interested in the results in equation 2 but is calculating a different probability in equation 1. These two equations can be related using Bayes' theorem. This relationship is best explained by creating an analogy to diagnostic testing.

A diagnostic test is interpreted in light of its sensitivity (the probability of a positive result given that the patient has the disease), its specificity (the probability of a negative result given that the patient does not have the disease), the prior probability of disease (usually the prevalence of disease in a population), and the predictive value of a positive test (the probability that the patient has the disease given that the test is positive). The probability of a positive result given that the patient does not have the disease is then 1 − specificity. The analogy of these terms to statistical testing is summarized in Table 3-5. These characteristics of a diagnostic test are related by the following equation:

$$p(\text{disease/positive test}) =$$

$$\frac{\text{prior probability} \times \text{sensitivity}}{[\text{prior probability} \times \text{sensitivity} + (1 - \text{prior probability}) \times (1 - \text{specificity})]}$$

(Equation 3)

One often orders a diagnostic test with the goal of obtaining a positive result, and one often performs a statistical test to reject the null hypothesis. Thus one can view a statistically significant result as analogous to a positive test, a nonstatistically significant result as analogous to a negative test, the presence of disease as analogous to the rejection of the null hypothesis, and the absence of disease as analogous to the truth of the null hypothesis. One can equate sensitivity with the statistical power of a test and specificity with 1 - p value. In essence, equations 1 and 2 can be related by Bayes' theorem by the following:

$$p(H_0 \text{ false}/ \text{ reject } H_0) =$$

$$\frac{\text{prob } (H_0 \text{ false}) \times \text{power}}{[\text{prob}(H_0 \text{ false}) \times \text{power} + \text{prob } (H_0 \text{ true}) \times \text{p value}]}$$

(Equation 4)

Table 3-5. Analogy Between Statistical Tests and Diagnostic Tests

Diagnostic Test	Statistical Test
Absence of disease	Null hypothesis correct
Presence of disease	Null hypothesis incorrect
Abnormal test (positive test)	Reject null hypothesis
Normal test result	Do not reject null hypothesis
Sensitivity	Power*
1 – specificity (false-positive rate)	p value
A priori probability of disease	A priori probability of the null hypothesis being incorrect
Predictive value of a positive test	Probability the null hypothesis is not correct when the study is positive ($p < 0.05$)

*The power of a statistical test is the probability of rejecting the null hypothesis when, in fact, the null hypothesis is incorrect.

where prob (H_0 false) denotes the a priori probability that the null hypothesis is false.

Just as we can determine the predictive value of a positive diagnostic test using the prior probability of disease, sensitivity, and specificity, so we can determine the probability that a statistically significant result is correct using the prior probability that the null hypothesis is false, the statistical power of a test, and the p value. Just as the positive predictive value of a diagnostic test is low if the prevalence of disease is low, the probability that a statistically significant result is correct is low if the prior probability of the null hypothesis being true is high. Use of equation 4 is a special type of statistical analysis called Bayesian statistical analysis and is not commonly used in biomedical literature. The reason for this is due to difficulties in determining the exact a priori probability and power. Nonetheless, a qualitative understanding of the principles of Bayesian statistics outlined above should prevent the misinterpretation of p values.

Understanding a Bayesian analysis can explain why two individuals may read the same study and come to different conclusions. As an example, suppose a study demonstrates that transfusion is associated with an increased recurrence rate of cancer in patients undergoing resection for colon cancer (p = 0.05). Assume that the study had a statistical power of 80%. Also assume that on the basis of previous data and animal models, blood banker A felt that the likelihood of an association between transfusion and cancer recurrence was only 0.05, while blood banker B felt that this likelihood was 0.9. Using equation 4, the probability that the study was correct according to blood banker B is $0.9 \times 0.8 / [0.9 \times 0.8 + 0.1 \times 0.05]$ = 0.99. The probability of the study being correct according to blood banker A is $0.05 \times 0.8 / [0.05 \times 0.8 + 0.95 \times 0.05]$ = 0.46. After examining the same study, blood banker B will be highly confident that transfusion has an adverse effect on cancer survival and blood banker A will remain unconvinced.

The use of Bayesian analysis in the previous example may strike the reader as not being objective. The final interpretation of a scientific study is markedly affected by one's a priori subjective bias as to whether or not the null hypothesis its true. On further consideration, however, one should note that the Bayesian analysis better reflects how decisions are made. If we are reasonably certain that the null hypothesis is false before an experiment, we need less evidence (a larger p value) to be comfortable rejecting the null hypothesis than if we are reasonably certain that the null hypothesis is true before an experiment. This is identical to diagnostic testing where we may remain unconvinced that a positive test indicates that the patient has a disease when the prevalence of the disease is low.

Use of Confidence Intervals Instead of p Values— A Solution to the Limitations of p Values

As noted above, the p value provides no information concerning the clinical significance of an observed "difference." A statistically significant p value may be associated with a clinically insignificant difference, and a statistically insignificant p value may be associated with a clinically significant difference. Suppose that groups A and B are being compared with respect to a variable (eg, hemoglobin). The measured difference in the variable between the two groups is a point estimate of the true difference. This point estimate is the best estimate of the true difference (the true difference is always unknown). If the study were to be repeated many times, however, each time the measured difference would vary. In order to address this variation, one can calculate an interval where 95% of the measured differences would lie. This is called a 95% confidence interval (95% CI). Thus, one may measure a mean difference in hemoglobin of 1.0 mg/dL between groups A and B. If the data are normally distributed and the standard error of the difference in means is 0.1 mg/dL, the 95% CI would include 0.8 mg/dL to 1.2 mg/dL. Methods for calculating 95% CIs are found in many texts.[11]

Many statisticians have advocated replacement of the p value with a 95% CI.[45] The advantage of this approach is that the 95% CI can be used to assess both clinical significance and statistical significance. The 95% CI can determine statistical significance in the following way. If the 95% CI contains a zero difference, then the results are not statistically significant. If the 95% CI does not contain a zero difference, as in the hemoglobin example above, then the results are statistically significant. Clinical significance can be assessed by determining the minimum difference deemed to be clinically important. If the 95% CI of the difference is entirely greater than this minimum important difference, then the difference is clinically significant. If the 95% CI of the difference is entirely less than the value of the minimum important difference, then the difference is not clinically significant. If the 95% CI contains points both greater than and less than the minimum clinically important difference, then no definite conclusion can be made. Nonetheless, trends may be suggested by noting if most of the 95% CI of the difference is either above or below the minimum clinically important difference. In the hemoglobin example above, if one viewed a hemoglobin difference of 1.5 mg/dL as the minimum clinically important difference, the results are statistically significant but clinically insignificant.

One can also determine clinical significance with a hypothesis by using a null hypothesis that states that two groups do not differ by more than a certain amount and attempt to disprove the null hypothesis. This is similar to the reformulated null hypothesis discussed in the section concerning establishing equivalency.

This type of analysis might disturb some investigators as not being scientific. After all, one must make a subjective decision as to what difference is clinically significant. Different knowledgeable individuals could have markedly different ideas on what is clinically important. Nonetheless, this subjectivity more accurately reflects reality. Ultimately, a new treatment or method must show enough difference from an old one to justify the costs, risks, or side effects. Dichotomization of results into p<0.05 or p>0.05 intended less than or greater than 0.05 is completely objective but ignores the highly relevant factor of how much difference is clinically significant. In this author's opinion, the p value is most valuable in preliminary investigations in which the clinical significance of a difference has yet to be determined. Studies iintended to modify medical practice are often better expressed by a CI rather than a p value.

In this context, it should be emphasized that the unqualified use of the term "significant" should be abolished from the medical lexicon.[59] One always needs to specify whether one is referring to statistically significant or clinically significant results.

p Values Cannot Be Used to Compare the Baseline Characteristics of Randomized Groups

As noted above, one method of avoiding confounding variables is randomization. Randomization is supposed to allocate patients or samples into groups without any bias. Thus, the distribution and values of any baseline variables (potential confounding variables) should be the same. In order to confirm this, the similarity of baseline characteristics must be established after randomization because random chance may not always result in an exactly equal distribution of baseline characteristics. In a review of how baseline characteristics are handled, Altman and Dore[20] noted that 58% of studies used hypothesis tests to determine if there were any differences in baseline characteristics after randomization.

It should be recognized that this is not a valid method for assessing similarity.[60] Assume that a researcher randomizes patients into two groups to study the effect of a new drug. The researcher wants to be assured that the two groups do not differ in hemoglobin levels prior to comparing the rate of successful treatments. If a statistical test is performed to determine whether there is a difference in hemoglobin levels, the null hypothesis states that the two groups are not different. The p value is the probability that the observed difference or a greater one could have arisen by chance when in reality there was no difference. Because the allocation to groups was random, any differences will by necessity be due to random chance. In essence, the statistical tests in this case are at best assessing whether or not randomization was correctly performed. Using a p value of 0.05 to establish significance, one should expect to find 5% of baseline comparisons to be statistically significant in a randomized trial.

Schultz et al,[21] however, found that of the randomized controlled studies published in prestigious obstetric journals, there were fewer statistically significant differences in baseline comparisons (2%) than expected (5%). Schultz et al[21] speculated that investigators, after performing superfluous statistical tests and finding statistical significance, deliberately withheld that information in order to increase the credibility of their reports. Faulty randomization could also have played a role in this lower-than-expected incidence of statistical differences.

The value of a baseline variable will, in general, not be exactly the same in the two groups. Any difference should be evaluated by considering the magnitude of the difference in the value of the variable and the strength of its association with the outcome being measured. Two groups may have a difference in a baseline variable that is not statistically significant yet can explain the difference in the outcome variable being measured. Similarly, there may be a statistically significant difference in a baseline variable that has no or little effect on the outcome variable being measured. An example taken from Altman[60] will illustrate this problem.

Assume that two treatments (A and B) are compared with mortality as the measured endpoint. Suppose that a specific risk factor doubles the probability of dying and that 25% of patients have this factor. There are 400 patients in this study, allocated to the two treatment groups by simple randomization. The results are displayed in Table 3-6. The risk factor is exactly balanced in this case and the mortality rates are 50% and 40% in treatments A and B respectively. This difference is not quite statistically significant (p = 0.06, chi square).

Now consider cases in which the risk factor is not exactly balanced between the two treatment groups, yet the difference is not quite significant at the p = 0.05 level. In the first of two examples (Table 3-7), there is an excess of the risk factor in treatment group A and in the second example (Table 3-8) an excess of the risk factor in treatment group B. In Table 3-7, the difference in mortality between the two groups is sta-

Table 3-6. Mortality in Two Treatment Groups With an Equal Distribution of a Risk Factor That Has a Prevalence of 25% and a Relative Risk of 2.0

	Treatment A	Treatment B	Total
Risk factor present	40/50 (80%)	32/50 (64%)	72/100 (72%)
Risk factor absent	60/150 (40%)	48/150 (32%)	108/300 (36%)
Total	100/200 (50%)	80/200 (40%)	180/400 (45%)

p = 0.06 for the difference in mortality

Table 3-7. Mortality in Two Treatment Groups With a Nonstatistically Significant Increase of a Risk Factor in Group A Where the Risk Factor Has a Prevalence of 25% and a Relative Risk of 2.0

	Treatment A	Treatment B	Total
Risk factor present	47/59 (80%)	26/41 (64%)	73/100 (73%)
Risk factor absent	56/141 (40%)	51/159 (32%)	107/300 (36%)
Total	103/200 (51.5%)	77/200 (38.5%)	180/400 (45%)

p = 0.015 for the difference in mortality
p = 0.05 for the difference in the distribution of the risk factor between treatment groups

tistically significant (p = 0.015 by chi-square testing). In Table 3-8, the difference between the two groups is only p = 0.19, which is not statistically significant. In both tables, the difference in the distribution of the risk factor is on the borderline of statistical significance (p = 0.05). Thus, the prevalence of the risk factor may vary as much as that noted in Tables 3-7 and 3-8 and yet not be statistically significant. Despite this lack of statistical significance, there is a marked effect on the p values.

In Altman and Dore's review,[20] 16% of the trials did not make any adjustment for a major difference in baseline characteristics. A major difference was defined as a subjective substantial difference in means or proportions, regardless of statistical significance. If a difference is noted in the baseline characteristics, one can adjust for this by using multivariate statistical modeling.[20] Sometimes a nonstatistical discussion might adequately address any differences in baseline characteristics.

Descriptive Statistics

The use of descriptive statistics is a part of statistical analysis that is frequently omitted or markedly abbreviated in statistical texts, perhaps because of its simplicity. The amount of data collected is usually too large to be fully presented in an

Table 3-8. Mortality in Two Treatment Groups With a Nonstatistically Significant Increase of a Risk Factor in Group B Where the Risk Factor Has a Prevalence of 25% and a Relative Risk of 2.0

	Treatment A	Treatment B	Total
Risk factor present	33/41 (80%)	38/59 (64%)	71/100 (71%)
Risk factor absent	64/159 (40%)	45/141 (32%)	109/300 (36%)
Total	97/200 (48.5%)	83/200 (41.5%)	180/400 (45%)

p = 0.19 for the difference in mortality
p = 0.05 for the difference in the distribution of the risk factor between treatment groups

article. The p value alone is insufficient to adequately report the results of a study because it merely states the results of hypothesis testing (ie, is the null hypothesis false?). Thus, one is forced to summarize data. This may be done graphically (eg, histograms) or by presenting a measure of the central tendency of the data and a measure of the variability of the data about this central tendency.

Most commonly, data are described by a mean and standard deviation (SD). This type of description, however, assumes that the data are normally distributed. If the data are not normally distributed, one can still calculate and report a mean and standard deviation; however, these numbers may be highly misleading.[7]

For example, one study compared two different methods of autologous blood recovery in reducing allogeneic red cell use in two groups of surgical patients. The authors reported that when method A was used, the mean allogeneic red cell use was 0.4 ± 0.8 unit (mean ± SD) per patient vs a mean allogeneic red cell use of 1.2 ± 1.0 units (mean ± SD; p<0.05) when method B was used. If the data were normally distributed, approximately 95% of the patients using method A would have received a number of allogeneic units within two standard deviations of the mean. In this case, 2 SDs = 1.6, so if the data were normally distributed, approximately 95% of the patients would have received between −1.2 and 2.0 units. Clearly, one cannot receive a negative number of units. Thus, the data are not normally distributed, virtually no information is conveyed by the SD, and the information presented is misleading. More important, one cannot interpret the statistically significant p value optimally. One can state that there is a difference between the two methods that is unlikely to be accounted for by chance alone, but one does not really know the magnitude of the difference. Therefore, one would have difficulty in deciding which method is better. Specifically, in the above example, one can see that method A resulted in a lower allogeneic blood use of 0.8 unit per patient on average. However, one does not know whether this difference was uniform for all of the patients studied or was the result of a difference in only one or a few patients. The latter information would be conveyed by an indication of the variability about the central tendency, and this variability must be described in terms that are appropriate for data that are not normally distributed.

In cases where data are not normally distributed, it is better to give a median and some percentiles (ie, the 25th and 75th percentiles).[11] Alternatively, one can give the interquartile range (the difference between the 25th and 75th percentiles).[11] For data that are highly skewed, a median gives a much better idea of the central tendency of the data than the mean. For some sets of data, particularly small sets, a range may be preferable.

The best way to determine if the data are normally distributed is by simple inspection of a histogram of the raw data. Verifying that most of the data are located within two standard deviations of the mean is also a useful check. There are more formal statistical tests for normality; however, they may be too sensitive for many purposes. Even if one does not have access to the raw data, certain simple checks are available. When all of the data must be greater than zero, a standard deviation of greater than one-half of the mean is a clue to the presence of nonnormality.[61] If the SD is only slightly greater than one-half of the mean, the data may be approximately normally distributed. The greater the SD is relative to one-half of the mean, however, the greater is the deviation from normality. Another check would be that the standard deviation should be approximately one-third of the range. Examples of this that occur in transfusion medicine include residual leukocyte counts after filtration, number of transfused units in a group of patients, and CD34 counts in progenitor cell collections.

Description of Paired Data

Sometimes measurements are made on the same individuals or samples before and after an event. In this type of experiment, a patient is used as his or her own control. One is interested only in the change in each individual. This is a useful type of experimental design that may have more power to detect a difference than using an unpaired analysis.

The type of statistical test used on paired data is different from that used on unpaired data. For normally distributed data, one would use a paired t test, and for dichotomous data, one would use McNemar's test. Usually, but not always,[7] the researcher performs the correct test. Problems frequently arise, however, when the data are described. Many times, the researcher will ignore the pairing when presenting the data. Moreover, in some instances, an investigator will entirely rely on the p value when it is of little interest.

An example illustrates this. Hemoglobin measurements were taken on a series of consecutive hysterectomy patients before preoperative autologous donation (PAD) and at admission.[26] One goal of the study was to determine the role of PAD in causing preoperative anemia. Patients were eligible if the hematocrit was not less than 33% and surgery was elective. A total of 123 patients was studied. Results are displayed in Table 3-9 using a mean and standard deviation. (The original publication did not present or analyze the data in this fashion for reasons noted below.)

Table 3-9. Hemoglobin Change From Preoperative Autologous Blood Donation in 123 Patients

Predonation Hemoglobin	Admission Hemoglobin	p Value
13.5 ± 1.5 mg/dL	11.8 ± 1.1 mg/dL	<0.000001

Lack of a Need for a t Test

If one is to perform a statistical test, a two-tailed paired t test is the correct test to perform. Nonetheless, this simple study illustrates a conceptual problem with statistical tests. That is, does one need a statistical test? The t test analyzes whether the donation of blood decreases hemoglobin over the next few weeks. Obviously, it does. One starts with a certain amount of blood in the body, removes approximately 10% of that blood, and in the absence of magic or divine intervention, one is clearly left with less blood in the patient than was present prior to donation. Proving that phlebotomy decreases hemoglobin with a t test should be of little interest. What most blood bankers want to know is how much the hemoglobin decreased by PAD. This is an estimation problem. In this case, the hemoglobin fell, on average, 1.7 mg/dL.

Nonoptimal Use of Descriptive Statistics

In addition to the average decrease in hemoglobin, the variability of this decrease is also important. Do all patients have a similar decrease in hemoglobin or is the decrease much larger for some patients than others? Assuming that hemoglobin levels and the difference in hemoglobin levels before and after PAD are normally distributed, this variability can be measured by the standard deviation. Unfortunately, the standard deviations given in Table 3-9 are measures of the variability of the hemoglobin levels of the patients in the study, rather than of the variability of the change in hemoglobin level resulting from the blood donation. In fact, the decrease in hemoglobin in the above study was 1.7 ± 1.4 mg/dL (mean ± SD). Stating results this way delineates the variability of the decrease in hemoglobin. Although, in this case, the standard deviation of the difference is not that much different than the standard deviation of the predonation and admission hemoglobin, in general, this is not the case.

One advantage of the experimental design in this study is that it is a paired study. The difference in hemoglobin is measured for each patient. This is a more powerful design as each patient serves as his or her own control. Presentation of the standard deviation as done above, however, ignores the pairing of the data and thus disregards important information.

Presentation of Results—Absolute vs Relative Risk

Suppose that an investigator compares two groups of patients and finds a statistically significant difference in a particular characteristic. Also suppose that he or she recognizes that the p value does not describe the magnitude of this difference. There are several methods to present this difference properly. The manner in which the difference is presented may affect how readers interpret the study.[62,63]

Differences may be represented as absolute or relative differences.[63] Suppose that p_i = the proportion of patients or samples in group i that have a certain characteristic. The absolute difference between two groups is $p_1 - p_2$. The relative difference is $(p_1 - p_2)/p_1$. (This should not be confused with an epidemiologic term called the relative risk, which is p_1/p_2.) The number of patients or samples needed to observe one unit of difference in the characteristic is $1/(p_1 - p_2)$. Statistically significant differences may be expressed in any or all of these ways. Several studies, however, have noted that given the same data, differences expressed as a relative difference are more likely to influence physicians' practices than the same information expressed as an absolute difference. Both absolute and relative differences were more likely to influence physicians' behavior than the same information presented as the number of patients needed in order to observe one difference in outcome.[62,63] Similar findings have been noted when such data were presented to patients as well.[64,65] Patients were more likely to desire therapy when the efficacy of the therapy was expressed in relative differences.

This finding should not be too surprising. The same 25% reduction may be reported for a study in which the event rates are 40% and 30% (a 10% absolute reduction) as for a study in which the event rates are 4% vs 3% (only a 1% absolute reduction). For events with a low probability, such as disease transmission from transfusion, there may be very large relative reductions in risk with very small absolute differences. For example, suppose that a study found that one groups of donors had twice the risk of transmitting hepatitis as a control group. For simplicity, assume that the rate of hepatitis B transmission is approximately 1/50,000 in the control population. Results can be reported as a relative risk of 2.0, or an absolute risk difference of 1/50,000 (1/25,000-1/50,000). Given that the manner in which the results are reported may affect how these results are viewed, it would seem reasonable to at least report both the relative and absolute risks.[62]

How to Prove That Something Is 100% Safe—An Exercise in Futility

Many studies are designed to describe the risk of an adverse outcome. If that outcome is unlikely to occur, the study may observe no adverse events. The interpretation of finding such a result may be difficult. Often, the occurrence of no events is viewed much differently than the occurrence of a few rare events. For example, a study of recipients of blood components from donors who later developed Creutzfeldt-Jakob disease (CJD) was recently reported.[66] No cases of disease transmission were noted. Had this report found even one case of disease transmission, the effects on transfusion practices and the blood bank community would be greatly different.

Studies reporting no adverse events (a zero numerator) must be carefully interpreted. In particular, the researcher needs to report a 95% confidence interval. A simple rule of thumb, "the rule of three," states that if none of n patients shows the event, the upper limit of the 95% confidence interval is $3/n$.[67] This rule of thumb is very accurate if n >30. For example, in the above study,[66] 179 recipients of blood components made from a donor who later developed CJD were followed and no cases of disease transmission were found. The 95% CI would extend to 3/179 = 1/60. If one is unsure of the incubation period of the disease after transfusion, one would be more interested in the fact that no disease was found in 41 long-term survivors (>5 years). The upper 95% CI is 3/41 = 1/13.7. Thus, in long-term survivors, the risk is likely to be anywhere from zero to 1/13.7. It should be obvious that many more patients would need to be followed if one wanted to be more certain that CJD is never transmitted by transfusion.

Similar problems arise in the study of the safety of lowering the transfusion trigger for platelets or red blood cells. One may not find any adverse outcomes, but this does not mean that they will never occur. Some early studies of the safety of autologous donation that reported no serious adverse outcomes were also based on small sample sizes. These studies may not have been large enough to detect the small but not insignificant risk of a severe reaction (1/17,000) reported in a larger series.[68]

Summary

Statistical analysis should be viewed as a type of mathematical model. Like other mathematical models, one must be constantly aware of the assumptions underlying the model as well as the precise meaning of various parameters and mathematical quantities (eg, the p value). Misunderstanding the meaning of the p value and suboptimal description of the data may cause errors in the interpretation of data. Use of statistics or statisticians as a "black box" that mysteriously yields the correct answer may provide a false sense of security and result in a failure to recognize some of these types of issues. The blood banker needs to be aware of the many hidden assumptions in statistical analysis so that he or she knows when to obtain statistical advice.

Acknowledgment

The author wishes to thank Girma Wolde-Tsadik, PhD, for his critical review of this manuscript.

References

1. Riggs DS. The mathematical approach to physiological problems. Cambridge, MA: MIT Press, 1963:1-5.
2. Riggs DS. Control theory and physiological feedback mechanisms. Baltimore: Williams and Wilkins, 1970:21.
3. Cohen JA, Brecher ME. Preoperative autologous blood donation: Benefit or detriment? A mathematical analysis. Transfusion 1995;35:640-4.

4. Kanter M. Transfusion-associated graft-versus-host disease: Do transfusions from second-degree relatives pose a greater risk than those from first-degree relatives? Transfusion 1992;32:323-7.
5. Lackritz EM, Satten Ga, Aberle-Grasse J, et al. Estimated risk of transmission of the human immunodeficiency virus by screened blood in the United States. N Engl J Med 1995;333:1721-5.
6. Schreiber GB, Busch MP, Kleinman SH, Korelitz JJ. The risk of transfusion-transmitted viral infections. N Engl J Med 1996;334:1685-90.
7. Kanter MH, Taylor JR. Accuracy of statistical methods in *Transfusion*: A review of articles from July/August 1992 through June 1993. Transfusion 1994;34:697-701.
8. Connett JE. Biostatistical red flags. Transfusion 1994; 34:651-3.
9. Easterbrook PJ, Berlin JA, Gopalan R, Matthews DR. Publication bias in clinical research. Lancet 1991;337: 867-72.
10. Dickersin K, Min YI, Meinert CL. Factors influencing publication of research results: Follow-up of applications submitted to two institutional review boards. JAMA 1992;267:374-8.
11. Altman DG. Practical statistics for medical research. London: Chapman and Hall, 1991.
12. Box GEP, Hunter WG, Hunter JS. Statistics for experimenters: An introduction to design, data analysis, and model building. New York: John Wiley & Sons, 1978.
13. Lilienfeld DE, Stolley PD. Foundations of epidemiology, 3rd ed. Oxford: Oxford University Press, 1994.
14. Kanter MH, Petz L. The validity of statistical analyses in the transfusion medicine literature with specific comments concerning studies of the comparative safety of units donated by autologous, designated, and allogeneic donors. Transfus Med 1995;5:91-5.
15. Kanter MH. The transfusion audit as a tool to improve transfusion practice: A critical appraisal. Transfus Sci 1998;19:69-81.
16. Eisenstaedt RS. Modifying physicians' transfusion practice. Transfus Med Rev 1997;270:961-6.
17. Vamvakas E, Moore SB. Perioperative blood transfusion and colorectal cancer recurrence: A qualitative statistical overview and meta-analysis. Transfusion 1993;33: 754-65.

18. Evans M, Pollock AV. Trials on trial: A review of trials of antibiotic prophylaxis. Arch Surg 1984;119:109-13.
19. Mosteller F, Gilbert JP, McPeek B. Reporting standards and research strategies for controlled trials: Agenda for the editor. Control Clin Trials 1980;1:37-58.
20. Altman DG, Dore CJ. Randomisation and baseline comparisons in clinical trials. Lancet 1990;335:149-53.
21. Schultz KF, Chalmers I, Grimes DA, Altman DG. Assessing the quality of randomization from reports of controlled trials published in obstetrics and gynecology journals. JAMA 1994;272:125-8.
22. Kasper SM, Gerlich W, Buzello W. Preoperative red cell production in patients undergoing weekly autologous blood donation. Transfusion 1997;37:1058-62.
23. Yamada AH, Lieskovsky G, Skinner DG, et al. Impact of autologous blood transfusions on patients undergoing radical prostatectomy using hypotensive anesthesia. J Urol 1993;149:73-6.
24. Heiss MM, Mempel W, Delanoff C, et al. Blood transfusion-modulated tumor recurrence: First results of a randomized study of autologous versus allogeneic blood transfusion in colorectal cancer surgery. J Clin Oncol 1994;12:1859-67.
25. Busch ORC, Hop WCJ, Haynck van Pependrecht MAW, et al. Blood transfusions and prognosis in colorectal cancer. N Engl J Med 1993;328:1372-6.
26. Kanter MH, van Maanen D, Anders KH, et al. Perioperative autologous blood donations before elective hysterectomy. JAMA 1996;276:798-801.
27. Ringel M. Labs assess transfusions. CAP Today 1995; 9:10.
28. Bowden RA, Slichter SJ, Sayers M, et al. A comparison of filtered leukocyte-reduced and cytomegalovirus (CMV) seronegative blood products for the prevention of transfusion-associated CMV infection after marrow transplant. Blood 1995;86:3598-603.
29. Wenz B. Leukocyte reduction. ABC Newsletter September 5, 1997.
30. Kruskall MS, Chambers LA, Pacini D, et al. Estimating the safety of autologous blood units available for transfusion to homologous recipients. Transfusion 1989;29:373-4.
31. AuBuchon JP, Dodd RY. Analysis of the relative safety of autologous blood units available for transfusion to homologous recipients. Transfusion 1988;28:403-5.

32. Bland JM, Altman DG. Correlation, regression, and repeated data. Br Med J 1994;308:896-7.
33. Kanter MH, Poole G, Garratty G. Misinterpretation and misapplication of p values in antibody identification: The lack of value of a p value. Transfusion 1997;37:816-22.
34. Yomtovian R, Laxarus HM, Goodnough LT, et al. A prospective microbiologic surveillance program to detect and prevent the transfusion of bacterially contaminated platelets. Transfusion 1993;33:902-9.
35. Bacterial contamination of platelet pools—Ohio, 1991. MMWR 1992;41:36-7.
36. Pocock SJ. Clinical trials: A practical approach. New York: Wiley, 1983:240-2.
37. Pocock SJ. Current issues in the design and interpretation of clinical trials. Br Med J 1985;290:39-42.
38. Starkey JM, MacPherson JL, Bolgiano DC, et al. Markers for transfusion-transmitted disease in different groups of blood donors. JAMA 1989;262:3452-4.
39. Glantz SA. Primer of biostatistics. New York: McGraw Hill, 1992:278-86.
40. Salim Yusuf D, Wittes J, Probstifield J, Tyroler HA. Analysis and interpretation of treatment effects in subgroups of patients in randomized clinical trials. JAMA 1991;266:93-8.
41. O'Brien PC, Shampo MA. Statistical considerations for performing multiple tests in a single experiment 6. Testing accumulating data repeatedly over time. Mayo Clin Proc 1988;63:1245-50.
42. Freiman JA, Chalmers TC, Smith H, Kuebler RR. The importance of beta, the type II error and sample size in the design and interpretation of the randomized control trial. N Engl J Med 1978;299:690-4.
43. AuBuchon JP. Lessons learned from decision analysis. Transfusion 1996;36:755-60.
44. Kolmogorov AN, Fomin SV. Introductory real analysis. New York: Dover Publications, 1970:13.
45. Braitman LE. Confidence intervals assess both clinical significance and statistical significance. Ann Intern Med 1991;114:515-7.
46. Ware JH, Antman EM. Equivalence trials. N Engl J Med 1997;337:1159-61.
47. Blackwelder WC. "Proving the null hypothesis" in clinical trials. Control Clin Trials 1982;3:345-53.
48. Dunnett CW, Gent M. Significance testing to establish equivalence between treatments, with special reference

to data in the form of 2X2 tables. Biometrics 1977;33: 593-602.
49. Leukocyte reduction for the prevention of transfusion-transmitted cytomegalovirus (TT-CMV). Association Bulletin 97-2. Bethesda, MD: American Association of Blood Banks, 1997.
50. Strauss RG. Practical issues in neonatal transfusion practice. Am J Clin Pathol 1997;107(Suppl 1):S57-S63.
51. Snyder EL. Component selection: The role of leukocyte reduction. In: Fridey JL, Simpson MB, eds. Component selection: Polemics and politics. Bethesda, MD: American Association of Blood Banks, 1996:69-90.
52. Landaw EM, Kanter M, Petz LD. Safety of filtered leukocyte-reduced blood products for prevention of transfusion-associated cytomegalovirus infection. Blood 1996;87:4910-9.
53. FDA blood panel finds fault with data suggesting that leukoreduction is equivalent to donor testing in preventing CMV. ABC Newsletter September 19, 1997.
54. The continuous infusion versus double-bolus administration of Alteplase (COBALT) investigators. A comparison of continuous infusion of alteplase with double-bolus administration for acute myocardial infarction. N Engl J Med 1997;337:1123-30.
55. Lurie P, Wolfe SM. Unethical trials of interventions to reduce perinatal transmission of the human immunodeficiency virus in developing countries. N Engl J Med 1997;337:853-6.
56. Ware JH, Mosteller F, Delgado F, et al. P values. In: Bailar JC, Mosteller F, comps. Medical uses of statistics, 2nd ed. Boston: New England Journal of Medicine Books, 1992:181-200.
57. Hirsch RP, Riegelman RK. Statistical operations: Analysis of health research data. Cambridge, MA: Blackwell Science, 1996.
58. Browner WS, Newman TB. Are all significant p values created equal? The analogy between diagnostic tests and clinical research. JAMA 1987;257:2459-63.
59. International committee of medical journal editors. Uniform requirements for manuscripts submitted to biomedical journals. JAMA 1993;269:2282-6.
60. Altman DG. Comparability of randomised groups. Statistician 1985;34:125-36.
61. Kanter MH. Statistics in transfusion medicine: A review of common errors. In: Fridey JL, Kasprisin CA, Cham-

bers LA, Rudmann SV, eds. Numbers for blood bankers. Bethesda, MD: American Association of Blood Banks, 1995:77-104.
62. Forrow L, Taylor WC, Arnold RM. Absolutely relative: How research results are summarized can affect treatment decisions. Am J Med 1992;92:121-4.
63. Naylor CD, Erluo C, Strauss B. Measured enthusiasm: Does the method of reporting trial results alter perceptions of therapeutic effectiveness? Ann Intern Med 1992;117:916-21.
64. Hux JE, Naylor CD. Communicating the benefits of chronic preventive therapy: Does the format of efficacy data determine patients' acceptance of treatment? Med Decis Making 1995;15:152-7.
65. Malenka DJ, Baron JA, Johansen S, et al. The framing effect of relative and absolute risk. J Gen Intern Med 1993;8:543-8.
66. Sullivan MT, Schonberger LB, Kessler D, et al. Creutzfeldt-Jakob disease (CJD) investigational lookback study (abstract). Transfusion 1997;37(Suppl):2S.
67. Hanley JA, Lippman-Hand A. If nothing goes wrong, is everything all right? Interpreting zero numerators. JAMA 1983;249:1743-5.
68. Popovsky MA, Whitaker B, Arnold NL. Severe outcomes of allogeneic and autologous blood donations: Frequency and characterization. Transfusion 1995;35:734-7.

In: Brecher ME, Busch MP, eds.
Research Design and Analysis
Bethesda, MD: American Association of Blood Banks, 1998

4

Human Subjects Research in the Blood Banking Environment: Institutional Review Board Approval and Informed Consent

Judith A. Hautala, PhD

SCIENTIFIC AND MEDICAL INVESTIGATORS are well aware of the need for human subjects research review and approval when conducting a clinical trial that involves exposing a human subject to a new drug, biologic, device, or procedure. In these instances, the clinical patient or healthy individual is expressly recruited for the study and a specific interaction with that person is central to the conduct of the study. The applicability of human subjects research review is less obvious when the study simply involves in-vitro laboratory or analytical use of samples, data, or information collected from normal volunteer blood donors. However, in the context of research conducted in blood banking and transfusion medicine, human subjects research regulations apply not only to clearly defined clinical studies, but also to any research that involves volunteer blood donors. Such research studies include:
- Collection of units/samples/data from research donors
- Use of materials or records obtained from healthy volunteer donors for purposes of transfusion (eg, units, samples, do-

---

Judith A. Hautala, PhD, Senior Director, Administration, American Red Cross, Holland Laboratory, Rockville, Maryland

nor records, records of testing for infectious disease markers, etc)
- Use of donor records to recruit donors for research studies
- Use of materials from donors for testing of experimental devices (eg, collection bags, filters, diagnostics, etc) or for testing of approved devices for unlicensed purposes
- Use of the donor in research conducted at the time of donation that is not directly associated with the donation

The interpretation and application of human subjects research regulations in the above situations are often not clear-cut. The regulations were written primarily to cover the more typical clinical study in which a patient or specifically recruited healthy individual is directly treated with the experimental product or procedure under investigation. Appropriate and consistent application of these same regulations to in-vitro laboratory research studies that constitute human subjects research only because they involve human blood samples can present quite a challenge to both investigators and reviewers. In addition, the ethical issues of confidentiality, linkage, right to know, etc, can be rather subtle, yet complex, with research studies involving materials or data provided by volunteer donors for purposes of transfusion, and not specifically for research.

The information presented in this chapter is designed to assist investigators in designing and obtaining approval for human subjects research studies conducted in the context of blood banking and transfusion medicine. The topics include: 1) a brief history of human subjects research regulations; 2) a decision-tree approach for evaluating whether human subjects review and approval are needed and, if so, what level of review is required; 3) the impact that human subjects review will have on study design; 4) the process of developing and administering informed consent; 5) ways to facilitate human subjects review and approval; and 6) several examples of specific human subjects research issues that are likely to arise in the context of blood banking.

Background

The underlying principles for the protection of human subjects involved in research are derived from three critical documents—the Nuremberg Code, the Declaration of Helsinki, and the Belmont Report. The Nuremberg Code, developed in the 1940s to assist the Nuremberg Military Tribunal in judging the human experiments conducted by the Nazis, established the basic standards still in use today governing the ethical conduct of research involving human subjects. The key provisions of the Code are voluntary consent, minimization of risk and harm, a favorable risk/benefit ratio, qualified researchers using appropriate study designs, and the subject's freedom to withdraw at any time. In 1964, the World Medical Association reinforced these principles in the Declaration of Helsinki, which also distinguished therapeutic from nontherapeutic research.

The first United States government regulations protecting the rights of human subjects in research became effective on May 30, 1974, although the National Institutes of Health had established Policies for the Protection of Human Subjects in 1966. Also in 1974, the National Commission for the Protection of Human Subjects of Biomedical and Behavioral Research was established to identify the basic ethical principles that should underlie human subjects research and to recommend guidelines for ensuring that those principles were adhered to. In 1979, the Commission released its Belmont Report elaborating three essential requirements for the ethical conduct of research involving human subjects: respect for persons, beneficence, and justice.

Respect for persons involves a recognition of the personal dignity and autonomy of individuals and the need to provide special protection for those persons with diminished autonomy. This concept underlies the need to obtain valid informed consent, which requires clear and adequate information about the study, full understanding by the individual of his or her role in the study, and full voluntary participation free from coercion and undue influence. *Beneficence* confers an obligation to protect the subject from harm by maximizing anticipated benefits and minimizing any potential risks. This concept requires consideration of benefits to society as well as to the individual and consideration of all possible harms, not just overt physical or psychological injury. *Justice* requires that procedures and criteria for the selection of research subjects be fair and that certain disadvantaged populations (eg, the institutionalized, mentally infirm, prisoners, etc) be involved only under defined conditions.

The Belmont Report also articulated a distinction between "practice" and "research" while recognizing that the distinction between a therapeutic regimen and a research study is often blurred. Medical or behavioral practice is defined as an intervention designed solely to provide diagnosis, preventive treatment, or therapy to an individual. In contrast, research is defined as an activity that tests a hypothesis, contributes to generalizable knowledge and is usually described by a formal protocol that sets forth study objectives and procedures to accomplish those objectives. Despite this distinction, the Report recognizes that experimental procedures do not necessarily constitute research and that practice and research can occur simultaneously.

In 1981, both the Department of Health and Human Services (DHHS) and the Food and Drug Administration (FDA) responded to the Belmont Report by making significant revisions to their human subjects research regulations. The DHHS regulations, which are contained in the *Code of Federal Regulations*, Title 45 CFR Part 46, were revised again in 1991 and at that time became the Federal Policy for the Protection of Human Subjects (sometimes known as the Common Rule). Under this federal policy, DHHS regulations apply to human subjects research that is conducted, supported, or otherwise subject to regulation by the DHHS and 15 other federal departments and agencies, including the Department of Defense, the Centers for Disease Control and Prevention, the Department of Energy, the Department of Education, and the National Science Foundation. FDA regulations for the protection of human subjects are found in Title 21 CFR Parts 50 and 56. These regulations apply to the use of human subjects in all research involving products regulated by the FDA, including clinical investigations that will be used to support requests for research and marketing permits for drugs, biologic products, medical devices for human use, food and color additives, or electronic products.

In certain instances, DHHS and FDA regulations may apply simultaneously to a given human subjects research study. The two sets of regulations are very similar and differ primarily in the mechanism used by the two agencies to ensure compliance. The FDA conducts inspections of research facilities to determine if an institution is in compliance with the regulations. The DHHS relies on a mechanism whereby institutions provide prior written assurance to the Office for Protection from Research Risks (OPRR) within DHHS that the research will be carried out in accordance with DHHS regulations. For most large biomedical research institutions, this assurance is provided by a single umbrella assurance approved by the OPRR, called a Multiple Project Assurance of Compliance (MPA). The specific contents of the MPA are negotiated between the institution and the OPRR, but, in general, if the institution receives any federal funding, the MPA can be expected to apply to all research involving human subjects conducted by the institution regardless of the source of funding for the specific project.

Under both DHHS and FDA regulations, an institution conducting or supporting human subjects research is required to establish an Institutional Review Board (IRB) with the authority to approve, require modification of, or disapprove all such research. The primary mission of an IRB is to ensure that research involving human subjects meets the highest ethical standards. This mission is carried out by reviewing all human subjects research protocols within its jurisdiction prior to their initiation and providing continuing review of each protocol on at least an annual basis. Institutional officials may not approve research if it has been disapproved by the IRB.

Criteria for IRB Review and Approval

When planning a research study that involves human subjects in any way, including as a source of material or data, an investigator must evaluate whether IRB review and approval are needed and, if so, what level of review is required. This is best accomplished by asking a series of questions.

Is the Proposed Study a Research Study?

To qualify as research under DHHS regulations, the study must be one that contributes to generalizable knowledge. In general, if the investigator intends to publish the results or otherwise present them in a public forum, the study is research. By contrast, if the same study is being performed entirely for internal quality control purposes or patient treatment and there is no intent to disseminate the results outside the institution, the study is not research and no IRB review is required. Nevertheless, in the case of quality control studies that involve human subjects, ethical review by the institution may be desirable. Under FDA regulations, any study whose results will be reported to the FDA in support of an application for a research or marketing permit is considered a clinical investigation and must undergo human subjects research review.

Does the Research Study Involve Human Subjects?

If there is an intervention or interaction with a living person that would not occur or would occur in some other fashion in the absence of the research study, then the study involves human subjects and IRB review is required. If the study does not involve such an intervention or interaction, but does generate data that can be linked to an individual in any way, then the study also involves human subjects and is subject to IRB review. For example, any research study using samples or data collected for transfusion that retain donor or the unit number or other identifier is considered human subjects research even if the research involves only physical processing of the blood sample or compilation or aggregate analysis of previously collected data. If, however, the identifier is removed prior to use in the research study, then the study is not human subjects research and is exempt from IRB review. Thus, the decision with regard to maintaining linkage between the sample and the donor is critical in establishing the need for IRB review. The ethical issues that must be addressed in deciding to unlink such a study are discussed below.

Certain research studies that are exempt from IRB review and approval have been explicitly described in the DHHS regulations. Of the six categories that are listed, the only category of general relevance to blood banking and transfusion medicine reads:

Research involving the collection or study of existing data, documents, records, pathological specimens, or diagnostic specimens, if these sources are publicly available or if the information is recorded by the investigator in such a manner that subjects cannot be identified, directly or through identifiers linked to the subjects.[1]

FDA regulations do not define any categories that are specifically exempt from IRB review. Therefore, all studies that involve human subjects in any way and are intended for submission to the FDA must undergo some level of IRB review and approval.

It should be noted that while exempt studies do not have to be reviewed by the IRB under federal regulations, most institutions require that these studies be submitted in some form to their IRB administrative structure in order that the investigator's conclusion that the study is exempt can be independently reviewed and verified.

What Risk Level Applies to the Human Subjects Research Study?

If a human subjects research study requires IRB review, the investigator must determine if the study qualifies as a minimal risk or risk study. Minimal risk studies are those in which the probability and magnitude of harm or discomfort anticipated in the research are not greater than those ordinarily encountered in daily life or during the performance of routine physical or psychological examinations or tests. This category has been interpreted to include the collection of blood for research in volumes of up to 525 mL as well as the in-vitro research use of units (in volumes of up to 525 mL), samples, and data collected from routine blood donors for the purpose of transfusion when linkage to the donor by the identifier is maintained. Minimal risk studies that do not qualify for expedited review (see below) must be reviewed and approved by a convened meeting of the IRB.

All other human subject research studies are considered risk studies and must be reviewed and approved by a convened meeting of the IRB. The risk category thus includes two procedures very common in the blood bank environment—standard apheresis and infectious disease testing. Any research study that uses material obtained by apheresis or that includes any type of infectious disease testing is considered a risk study. It has been proposed to the DHHS that research involving the collection of blood components by standard apheresis be considered minimal risk and added to the expedited review list, but the fate of this proposal is unknown. The OPRR has, however, recently indicated that infectious disease testing does not a priori mean that the research should be in the risk category. If the infectious disease testing is performed as part of standard clinical or blood center practices on samples that are subsequently used for research unrelated to such testing, the research need not be classified in the risk category because of the performance of those tests.

If the Study Is Minimal Risk, Does It Qualify for Expedited Review?

Some, but not all, research that falls into the minimal risk category is eligible for expedited review. Under the expedited review procedure, the IRB chairperson or other qualified IRB member reviews the application and may either approve it or determine that it requires review at a convened meeting of the IRB.

The types of research eligible for expedited review are listed in the *Federal Register* by the DHHS[2] and the FDA[3] and are referred to in 45 CFR 46.110 and 21 CFR 56.110. The current Expedited Review list includes the following categories especially relevant to blood banking and transfusion medicine research studies.

1. *Collection of blood samples by venipuncture, in **amounts not exceeding 450 mL** in an 8-week period and no more often than two times per week, from subjects 18 years of age and older and who are in good health and not pregnant.*[2] Note that the volume of 450 mL is included in the wording of the regulations and can only be changed by the DHHS. Therefore, the collection of blood for research in volumes exceeding 450 mL must undergo full IRB review even though many facilities collect more than 450 mL in a standard blood donation. However, the OPRR has concluded that a study may be eligible for expedited review even though the volume of donated

blood is greater than 450 mL, as long as the donation was made for transfusion purposes and the volume of blood donated is not altered by the research protocol.
2. *The study of existing data, documents, records, pathologic specimens, or diagnostic specimens.*[2] Current DHHS policy defines "existing" as units/samples/data collected prior to the research for a purpose other than the proposed research, including samples collected in research and nonresearch activities. Therefore, units/samples/data that are obtained for a purpose other than research (such as transfusion) cannot be considered existing if any portion is collected after the date on which the research project begins. Thus, expedited review would only apply to research with blood, blood components, samples, or donor records that were already available in their entirety at the time the project begins.
3. *Research on drugs or devices for which an investigational new drug exemption or an investigational device exemption is not required.*[2] Thus, expedited review applies only to devices that are either substantially equivalent to an existing device [510(k) devices] or are otherwise exempted from investigational device regulations.

A revised expedited review category list is under public comment at the time of this writing. Several of the proposed revisions are of particular interest to the blood bank and transfusion medicine community including: 1) collection of blood by fingerstick (and perhaps earstick), not just venipuncture, 2) collection of blood in amounts up to 525 mL, and 3) research involving prospectively collected identifiable residual specimens, discarded specimens, data, documents, and records. No date for implementation of the final revisions has been announced.

Impact of Human Subjects Research Regulations on Study Design

If an investigator concludes that a planned research study is subject to human subjects research regulation and IRB review, this can affect several important areas of study design including linkage, provision of confidentiality, communication of results to subjects, need for reconsent for future studies, origin of source materials, recruitment methods, and administration of informed consent.

Linkage

Given the profound effect that linkage has on the need for human subjects review, investigators should give careful consideration to the importance of maintaining linkage in their studies. If the validity and worth of the study results are not significantly enhanced by linkage, it may be best to design the study in an unlinked manner. Even if the investigator believes that the results might lead to a desire to obtain additional information about or recontact specific subjects, it may be preferable to run the initial phase in an unlinked manner. If interesting results are obtained, then a more extensive linked study can be designed in which the subject population is clearly identified and full informed consent is obtained.

However, in deciding to unlink a study, the investigator should give careful consideration to whether or not the information to be generated is of sufficient importance to the subject that an unlinked study would be unethical. This is of particular relevance when information concerning the possible health status of the subject likely will be generated. The ethical questions surrounding whether the information is of sufficient accuracy to be of clinical relevance, whether there is any action that can be taken based on the information, the subjects' right to know that the information is being generated, etc, can be very complex. The ethical issues associated with linkage are one of the reasons that many institutions require that exempt studies (which are often exempt only because they are unlinked) must be submitted to the IRB administrative structure for confirmation that an unlinked study is ethically appropriate.

Confidentiality

Because the confidentiality of study results is so central to ethical human subjects research, investigators must give careful thought to how confidentiality will be ensured for a linked study. Specific, proactive safeguards should be designed and implemented rather than making the perhaps naive assumption that no outside parties will have access to the study records.

Communication of Results to Subjects

The obligation to notify subjects of significant results from the research is an important aspect of the ethical conduct of human subjects research. The notification provisions of a study, however, must be designed with a clear eye to various ethical issues. For example, the investigator must ask whether the information will be of true value to the subject or cause undue alarm. In addition, an ethical decision must be made whether the investigator has the right and obligation to decide whether the subject receives certain information or whether the subject should be given the right to make that decision. Also a consideration is whether the subject should be given the right to decide *not* to be informed if the investigator's scientific and medical judgment is that the subject should be informed. Resolving these issues must be given serious attention during design of a human subjects research protocol.

Consent for Future Testing

Research studies associated with blood banking may often involve the use of stored samples or the creation of a specific repository related to marrow, progenitor cell, and cord blood donations. In the design of linked studies using human blood or tissue samples collected in the past, careful consideration must be given to whether the subject should have been given the right to specifically consent to having new tests performed on their samples. If the samples were collected as part of blood center activities for purposes of transfusion or creation of a clinical repository, the OPRR has interpreted the regulations to stipulate that no research studies should be done with those samples unless informed consent for the specific studies has been obtained or unless the IRB waives the requirement for informed consent (see below). If samples are collected into a repository as part of a research study, the investigator should provide the subjects with a clear explanation of the conditions under which future testing may be performed. The subject may be asked to consent to all future testing as a requirement to be included in the original study or may be given a set of alternative choices ranging from denying the right to perform any future testing to requesting that they be recontacted in the future and allowed to make a decision about the testing. The incorporation of such choices may be the most ethically appropriate design but will require a significant amount of record-keeping and follow-up.

Origin of Source Materials

Consideration of human subjects research regulations may have an important impact on the particular source materials used for a study. For most in-vitro studies with blood or blood components, it is often operationally simpler to use material collected for transfusion. However, when one considers the issues of linkage, informed consent, etc, it may be preferable in certain instances to use material from donors recruited specifically for the research project. Careful consideration of these issues prior to the design of the research study will facilitate IRB review and prevent delays in implementation.

Recruitment and Informed Consent Administration

Although the most important aspects of human subjects research regulations deal with treatment of subjects during the project, recruitment methods and conditions for administering informed consent are also scrutinized by IRBs. In particular, the subjects being approached should not be in a situation that would either impair their ability to make an objective decision or would place them in a position where they might feel they have an obligation to cooperate with the requesting investigator. Recruitment and consent should be administered as far in advance as practical and the conditions and timing for obtaining informed consent should be determined primarily by the rights and welfare of the subjects, not by the needs or convenience of the investigator.

Informed Consent

As a general rule, each human subject participating in a research study that is classified as either minimal risk or risk study must give his or her informed consent to that participation. However, under special circumstances, an IRB may waive informed consent for a minimal risk study. Examples where such a waiver might be appropriate are described below. If informed consent is required, the investigator is responsible for ensuring that the subject is fully informed and understands the potential risks and benefits of participation in the research, the exact procedures that will be performed during the research, all requirements for compliance (ie, taking medication, keeping follow-up appointments, etc) on the part of the subject, and any other information relevant to the subject's decision to participate. The subject must be given this information and allowed to make his or her decision in a setting that is free from coercion or the appearance of coercion.

Written Consent Forms

The written consent form, which serves to document the consent process, must embody all of the basic elements of informed consent outlined below. The prospective subject or his or her legally authorized representative must be given adequate opportunity to read the consent document (or have it read to him or her), and it is the investigator's responsibility to ensure that the prospective subject is fully informed of the risks and benefits of participation in the research at the time consent is obtained. The consent document must be signed and dated by the subject or his or her representative and the investigator/designee at the time consent is given and a copy given to the subject. The investigator must ensure that the original signed and dated copy of the informed consent is maintained in a manner consistent with the degree of confidentiality required for the study. Informed consent documents must be retained by the investigator for at least 3 years after completion of the study.[4]

One of the most common reasons for a delay in IRB approval of a protocol is an inadequate or poorly written consent form. The consent form should be a statement addressed to the subject and is best worded in the second person using language the subject can understand. This includes using short sentences and simple words, avoiding scientific or medical terms as much as possible, providing lay definitions for those terms that must be included, and providing translations into other languages for subjects who do not understand English. Consent forms must be geared to a reading level appropriate for the proposed subject population and should generally be directed at no more than an eighth-grade reading level. After completing an informed consent document, it is often useful to test it for understandability with one or two "mock subjects," such as high school students, prior to submitting it to the IRB.

Essential Elements of Informed Consent

A written consent form should include all of the following that apply.

1. *General purpose of the study.* The document must make clear the research nature of the study and the knowledge that the investigator seeks to obtain from the study. Use language such as, "We hope to learn...". If appropriate, note that the study will be testing for "safety" and/or "effectiveness."

2. *Invitation to participate.* This can be combined with the purpose of the study in language such as, "You are invited to participate in a study of...". The invitation must be explicit and must communicate that there is a choice to be made and that research is involved.

3. *Why and how the subject was selected.* Use language such as, "because you are a healthy adult," or "because you have asthma," or "because you have relatives with a specific disease..."etc. This inclusion of subject criteria helps the subject assess the nature and importance of his or her participation. If the statement of the purpose of the study indicates the subject population, it need not be repeated. Indicate the expected number of participants in the study, eg, "You will be one of 20 participants...".

4. *Procedures to be followed and duration of the subject's participation.* Describe the procedures to be followed, how long they will take, and their frequency. If it is not clear from the description of the procedures, indicate the total duration of the subject's participation in the study. If applicable, randomization and use of placebos should be disclosed and explained. If any of the procedures or devices are experimental, they should be identified as such.
5. *Discomforts and inconveniences.* Describe the discomforts and inconveniences that the subject might reasonably expect.
6. *Side effects and risks.* Describe any side effects that may result from the study and the likelihood and magnitude of harm from those side effects. Explain the risks associated with the study that depart from the risks associated with the established and accepted methods necessary to meet the subject's needs, including any possibility of physical, psychological, or social injury.
7. *Benefits to the subject or others.* Describe any benefits to the subject or others that might reasonably be expected from the study. The suggestion of a benefit to the subject can be a strong inducement to participation and, therefore, such statements must be limited to substantial and likely benefits. If the benefits to certain subjects are different from the benefits to other subjects, this must be made clear. Claims should not be made that emphasize the effectiveness of a study drug or procedure. If there is no direct benefit to the subject, this should be explicitly stated.
8. *Standard treatment withheld or alternative procedures available.* If any standard treatment is being withheld, this must be disclosed. If there are any alternative procedures that might be appropriate and advantageous to the subject, they must be described. "Appropriate and advantageous" must be interpreted in terms of standard practice of care and not by the investigator's personal judgment alone. In the volunteer blood donation environment, explain if there are any changes in the standard donation process.
9. *Confidentiality.* State the measures, if any, used to maintain the confidentiality of records identifying the

subject's participation in the study. If data obtained from the subject's participation will be made available to any person or organization other than the subject, the investigator, and the investigator's staff, describe the person or agencies to whom information will be furnished, the purpose of the disclosure, and the nature of the information to be furnished. Studies conducted to support an investigational new drug (IND) application, an investigational device exemption (IDE) application, or a premarket approval application must indicate to the participant that the FDA may have access to the records as part of their review.

10. *Costs or payments.* If there might be additional cost to the subject due to participation in the study, disclose that possibility. If the subject will receive payment for participation, describe and state the amount, including any provision for proration if subject does not complete the study. Payment must be reasonable and not coercive. If subjects receive services or treatment at a lower cost than would be charged nonsubjects, the reduction in cost must be disclosed.

11. *Treatment and compensation available in the event of a research-related injury.* For studies in the risk category, explain what compensation and/or medical treatment, if any, will be available to the subject in the event of physical injury as a direct result of participation in the study. Provide a contact name and phone number for reporting a research-related injury and for obtaining further information concerning treatment and compensation. No exculpatory language waiving the subject's legal rights or releasing anyone associated with the study from liability for negligence is permitted.

12. *Reasons for termination by investigator.* State explicitly under what conditions the subject's participation in the study may be terminated by the investigator without the subject's consent (eg, failure to follow instructions, cancellation of study, inability to collect a sample, etc).

13. *Voluntary nature of participation and freedom to withdraw.* Explicitly state that participation is voluntary using language such as, "Your decision whether to participate is entirely voluntary and will not change or

influence your future association (treatment, employment, if applicable, etc). If you decide to participate, you are free to withdraw at any time without harm to your rights or future relations." or "If significant new findings develop during the study that may alter your willingness to participate, you will be notified of those findings."

14. *Contacts for further information.* Provide a name and phone number for individual(s) whom the subject should contact if he or she has further questions about the research project or research subject's rights.
15. *Agreement to participate.* There are several approaches to the language expressing the subject's decision to participate. For example, "My signature indicates that I have read this consent form, been given an opportunity to ask questions about the information provided, and voluntarily decided to participate in this research. I have been told about the potential risks of participation and my option to withdraw at any time without penalty." If someone other than the subject is giving consent (eg, parents), the suggested language should be changed to: "My signature indicates that I have read this consent form, been given an opportunity to ask questions about the information provided, and voluntarily decided to permit_____ to participate in this research." Children who are capable of understanding the process must be given a simplified version of the consent form and an opportunity to assent to participate.
16. *Signatures.* There must be space for the signature and date of signature for the subject, the investigator or his or her designee, and any witness. If the subject's representative (eg, parent) is signing, there should be space for the signatory to indicate his or her relationship to the subject.

Although the above elements cover all the requirements for informed consent under federal law, there may be other elements of consent required by the IRB or added by an investigator. Investigators should also determine if there are any applicable state laws or regulations that impose additional requirements on the informed consent process.

Administration of Informed Consent

It is the responsibility of the investigator or his or her designee to ensure that informed consent is administered in a manner that promotes full understanding, minimizes the potential for coercion or undue influence, and allows the subject sufficient time and opportunity to consider thoughtfully whether he or she wishes to participate. If the information concerning the study is complex, the investigator should consider the use of informational brochures, audiovisual aids, tests of the information presented, and/or independent consent advisors. For both complex studies and ones that may expose the subject to a high degree of risk or discomfort, the investigator should attempt to provide a reasonable period of time between providing information about the study and obtaining consent. This will allow the subject to consider thoroughly the advantages and disadvantages of participation and allow him or her time to discuss the study with family and friends.

In situations in which the intended study population is known to not be fluent in English, a translated version of the consent form should be made available. For all other instances where the participant is not fluent in English, a translator must be provided. The use of a translator should be documented on the consent form and the translator should sign the form.

The investigator must give each subject or his or her representative a copy of the signed consent form. Having a copy of the form helps the subject to maintain continued understanding of his or her involvement in the research and can help to avoid problems should the subject forget that he or she has been informed previously of a risk or discomfort. It also assists the subject in recognizing differences between his or her actual experience and what was expected and contributes to preserving a good relationship between the investigator and the subject.

Facilitating the IRB Review Process

The best way for investigators to facilitate the IRB review process is to take the time to fully understand the human subjects research requirements prior to both designing the study and submitting the application for review. This small degree of extra effort on the part of the investigator will greatly improve the efficiency of the IRB approval process and also reduce frustrations on the part of the investigator, IRB members and IRB administrators. Investigators should learn to develop and evaluate their study designs not only from the point of view of scientific rigor but also with regard to the ethical treatment of human subjects. In addition to incorporating into the study design the specific elements described above, the investigator should review the entire study from the perspective of the human subject. This review should evaluate whether the study protects the rights, integrity, and autonomy of the subjects; provides the subjects with complete and accurate information before and after the study; and is sensitive to diverse religious, cultural, and ethical backgrounds. Incorporating these aspects into the study design from the beginning will help prevent often cumbersome modifications in response to IRB comments. Investigators should also develop their informed consent documents with careful adherence to the elements of informed consent described above and in the federal regulations. Deficiencies in the informed consent document are the single most common reason for a delay in IRB approval.

In order to provide IRB members with the information necessary to evaluate a proposed study, the documents prepared for IRB submission must include more than simply a scientific explanation of the study. Although the complete scientific protocol can be provided as an attachment, the documents must primarily address factors that are important for evaluating the degree to which the rights of human subjects are being protected. The most important elements are: 1) a clear, concise description of the purpose and specific aims of the study; 2) a clear rationale for the number and type of subjects involved; 3) a complete description of the procedures involving human subjects along with their possible risks and benefits; and 4) a thorough discussion of both linkage and confidentiality. IRB submissions that are prepared without a purposeful effort to identify, analyze, and address issues relevant to the ethical treatment of human subjects have a high probability of requiring significant modifications before approval is granted. It is also important to remember that not all members of an IRB have been trained scientifically or medically. Each IRB must contain lay members and it is important to communicate clearly to them as well.

Human Subjects Research Issues Relevant to Blood Banking

Research With Materials or Data Collected for Purposes of Transfusion

A significant percentage of the human subjects research conducted in the context of blood banking and transfusion medicine does not fit the typical definition of clinical research. Rather, these studies involve in-vitro laboratory experiments or data analyses using materials or records obtained from human subjects for purposes of clinical practice (ie, transfusion) rather than research. Because these studies embody significant overlap between research and clinical practice, it is often complicated to ensure appropriate and yet not overly burdensome human subjects review. Although the simplest approach would be to conduct unlinked studies and thus be exempt from IRB review, it may not be possible to do so in every instance due either to ethical considerations or to FDA requirements relative to tracking all units collected for transfusion. Therefore, it is useful to develop standard procedures for the review of these protocols.

For example, if an in-vitro laboratory research study is conducted in a linked fashion with a small number of samples diverted from transfusion over a period of several weeks, it is not practical to obtain informed consent from all donors when only an occasional unit will be diverted. Therefore, in these cases, it would be appropriate to request the IRB to grant a waiver of informed consent providing that there is no change in the routine blood donation process and no potential to generate information of personal significance to the donor. DHHS regulations permit the waiver of informed consent by the IRB if the following criteria are met:
- The research in its entirety does not involve greater than minimal risk.
- It is not practical to conduct the research without the waiver/alteration.

- Waiving informed consent will not adversely affect the subjects' rights and welfare.
- Pertinent information about the research will be provided to subjects at the conclusion of the research, if appropriate.

FDA regulations do not permit the waiver of informed consent per se, but only a waiver of the documentation of informed consent. Therefore, for studies intended for submission to the FDA, the IRB could be asked to approve a process whereby all donors whose units might be involved in the research study would receive an information sheet about the study at the time of donation and be allowed to decline participation, but there would not be a requirement for a signed consent. The FDA itself, however, can grant a full waiver of informed consent.

If an investigator intends to conduct numerous studies over time involving in-vitro laboratory experiments using blood or blood components obtained for purposes of transfusion or data analyses utilizing donor records, it may be appropriate to prepare a standing protocol covering such studies and submit each new study as an amendment. Each amendment could then be approved by an expedited review procedure including the waiver of informed consent. Each new study amendment would have to involve no change in the routine donation or data collection process and generate no information of potential clinical significance to the donor. For example, samples donated for purposes of transfusion could not be used in a linked fashion for performing sensitive genetic testing without submitting a separate protocol and perhaps obtaining full informed consent.

Stored Samples Collected for Purposes of Transfusion Constitute a Repository

The OPRR views stored blood and blood component samples that were originally collected for purposes of transfusion and that retain the unique identifiers as a repository similar to the various tissue repositories that have been developed for use in cancer research. If samples from such a repository are provided to outside investigators in a completely unlinked fashion with no potential for linkage by anyone in the future, then the collection facility may submit to its IRB a standing protocol to cover such distributions, adding each new study as an amendment. Such a standing protocol could include only studies that do not generate genetic or any other information of potential clinical significance to the donor. If repository samples are provided to outside investigators in a linked fashion, then IRB review and approval are required for each study. The level of risk and level of review will depend on the study to be performed.

Each distribution from the repository to an outside investigator must be covered by a Recipient Investigator Agreement with the outside institution containing the following language.

> Recipient acknowledges that the conditions for use of this research material are governed by the [Institution] IRB in accordance with DHHS regulations at 45 CFR 46. Recipient agrees to comply fully with all such conditions and to report promptly to the [Institution] any proposed changes in the research project and any unanticipated problems involving risks to subjects or others. Recipient remains subject to applicable State or local laws or regulations and institutional policies which provide additional protections for human subjects. This research material may only be utilized in accordance with the conditions stipulated by the protocol approved by the [Institution] IRB. Any additional use of this material requires prior review and approval by the [Institution] IRB and where appropriate, by an IRB at the recipient site.[5]

Research Requiring a Device Determination

Research studies associated with blood bank operations often involve the testing of new experimental devices such as bags and filters or diagnostic tests using blood samples obtained for either research or transfusion. Many of these studies are intended for submission to the FDA and therefore qualify as clinical investigations subject to human subjects research review. If the device is a diagnostic product intended for use in testing another regulated product, an approved 510(k) device, or a device covered by an IND approval or IDE, then no separate IRB device determination is required. In all other instances, the IRB must make a determination as to whether the device presents a significant or insignificant risk. If the study itself is eligible for expedited review, then the device determination can also be expedited. If the IRB determines that the device is a "significant risk" device, then the sponsor must obtain an IDE before the study can proceed.

Collaborative Research With Other Institutions

Many research studies conducted by blood bank investigators are collaborative endeavors that involve the use of blood components collected at a blood center for the experimental treatment of patients in a collaborating hospital. If both institutions have an IRB and human subjects are involved at both institutions (ie, donors at the blood center and patients at the hospital), then the entire study must be approved by both IRBs. If both institutions have an IRB and if *all* human subjects involvement takes place at only one institution, then an IRB cooperative agreement can be established. Such an agreement allows the IRB of the institution that is not directly involved with the human subjects to accept review by the other institution's IRB. IRB cooperative agreements must be developed by the respective IRB administrative offices and, if the project is federally funded, approved by the OPRR. For federally funded projects where only one of the collaborating institutions has an OPRR-approved MPA, the MPA institution can obtain an interinstitutional amendment in which the collaborating non-MPA institution ensures that it will comply with DHHS regulations under the terms of the collaborating institution's MPA. This allows the MPA institution's IRB to review and approve the collaborative research project.

FDA regulations do not provide any explicit mechanisms covering review of collaborative projects. Therefore, any human subjects research conducted under FDA regulations must be reviewed by the IRB of each institution where human subjects are involved directly in the research.

Progenitor Cell and Cord Blood Banking

The establishment of either a hematopoietic progenitor cell or cord blood bank in a research setting presents a number of interesting ethical challenges in terms of informed consent.

For cord blood banks, one of the key questions is whether consent should be obtained pre- or postnatally. Postnatal consent is certainly the simpler alternative in that consent can be solicited only from those mothers whose cord blood has been collected. When using postnatal consent, the cord blood sample would be collected without consent and then the mother would be approached before leaving the hospital with a request for her consent to storage and testing. This approach would require an IRB waiver of informed consent for collection of the sample and provisions for discarding the sample if the mother did not consent to storage and testing. The primary ethical concern with postnatal consent is the ability of the mother to make a calm, reasoned decision about something as complex as storage, use, and future testing of her infant's cord blood sample in the often emotionally charged atmosphere existing during the first hours after birth. Given the trend toward releasing mothers as rapidly as possible from the hospital, there will not always be the opportunity to wait even 24 hours before approaching the mother for consent. There is also concern that the mother could feel a high level of gratitude toward the hospital staff and therefore be subject to undue influence relative to consent.

Prenatal consent through obstetricians' offices is clearly preferable in terms of the opportunity to fully explain the process to the mother, to give her the opportunity to discuss it with her doctor and family, and to allow her to weigh the alternative of having her infant's cord blood sample stored in a commercial bank that would preserve it for her own family's use. The disadvantage is that only a small percentage of the mothers whose consent is obtained prenatally will have their infant's cord blood sample collected and stored due to the fact that cord blood bank staff are generally available at limited times in a given hospital. In addition, there is concern that enrolling only mothers who use private obstetricians will not provide the minority representation desired in a publicly available cord blood bank. A compromise solution such as providing prenatal *information* through obstetricians' offices and clinics, but obtaining postnatal *consent* should also be considered. Deciding when to obtain consent is thus a key element in the design of any research study involving establishment of a cord blood bank.

As new genetic and infectious disease tests become available, it will be important to perform these tests on previously banked progenitor cell and cord blood samples before their use in transplantation. Therefore, in obtaining informed consent for such cell banking, it is important to allow the donor (or the mother in the case of cord blood banks) to choose whether to have such unspecified future testing performed and, if it is performed, whether to be notified of the results. To provide the subject with full autonomy in making this decision, a series of options could be presented, such as:
1) Granting permission for future genetic or other testing and requesting to be notified of the results and provided information about those results.
2) Granting permission for future genetic or other testing and requesting not to be notified of the results.
3) Denying permission for future genetic or other testing.
4) Requesting to be informed before any future genetic or other testing is performed to be given the opportunity to permit or decline such testing, and, if the testing is permitted, to be allowed to choose whether to be informed of the results.

Conclusion

As blood banking moves into the 21st century, there will be an increasing level of sophistication in the technologies, instrumentation, and devices employed as well as in the advanced therapeutic products that can be developed from blood. This will mean an increasing emphasis on research and an increasing need to conduct studies that comply with human subjects research regulations. The information contained in this chapter is intended to serve as a "user-friendly" guide for accurately assessing the need for human subjects review; designing studies that comply with the regulations; facilitating the review and approval process; and establishing efficient, standardized mechanisms for the design, review, and approval of study categories that appear repeatedly in the context of blood bank research.

References

1. Code of federal regulations. Title 45 CFR Part 46, Section 101(b)(4). Washington, DC: US Government Printing Office, 1996.
2. Department of Health and Human Services. Research activities which may be achieved through expedited review procedures set forth in HHS regulations for protection of human subjects research; notice. Fed Regist 1981;46:8392.
3. Food and Drug Administration. Protection of human research subjects; clinical investigations which may be reviewed through expedited review procedures set forth in FDA regulations; notice. Fed Regist 1981;46:8980.
4. Code of federal regulation. Title 45 CFR Part 46, Section 115(b). Washington, DC: US Government Printing Office, 1996.
5. Issues to consider in the research use of stored data or tissues. November 7, 1997. Rockville, MD: Office for Protection from Research Risks, 1997.

In: Brecher ME, Busch MP, eds.
Research Design and Analysis
Bethesda, MD: American Association of Blood Banks, 1998

5

The Publication of Research Results

Jeffrey McCullough, MD

THE SUCCESS OF A research project and, ultimately, the ability to get the results published are influenced substantially by the type and amount of planning that is done. It is generally advisable not to rush into a new project but to take time to carefully think through the project and develop specific plans. While this might seem to be an obvious piece of advice or an ineffective use of time, it is important because it can avoid many problems, help to channel effort, and become a useful tool in gaining financial support for the project. This planning effort is usually also beneficial when the results are written for publication. Examples of steps or issues that may be considered in planning a research project and that may influence the "publishability" of the results of the project are briefly summarized in this chapter.

Planning the Research Project

Define the Reasons for Conducting the Study

It should be possible to rather concisely describe the reasons for carrying out the proposed study. These reasons should be

---

Jeffrey McCullough, MD, Department of Laboratory Medicine and Pathology, University of Minnesota, Minneapolis, Minnesota

put into written form. The process of writing the reasons for the study requires the investigator to document what is known or not known about the subject, including an analysis of existing data or information on the subject. This process thus involves literature review and a thoughtful examination of existing information leading to a rationale for the proposed study. Describing this information enables the investigator to provide a solid foundation for carrying out the study, and the material becomes the basis of the introduction to the report of the study. Thus, in carrying out a careful examination of what is known about the proposed subject and using these data or this information to develop a written description of why the study is necessary, the investigator has essentially a draft of the introduction for the final manuscript.

Define the Purpose of the Study

When the reasons for carrying out the study have been defined, there is a natural flow of ideas into defining the purpose of the study. Before undertaking any research project, it is essential for the investigator to clearly state the reason for the study. It should be possible to complete the sentence, "The purpose of this study is to ...". This may then become the ending statement of the introduction section of the manuscript. Stating the purpose of the study helps to focus the investigators and provides a reference point as the study unfolds so that the progress of the study can be measured against the original idea of the reasons for the study. This step also will form the basis for many of the decisions that have to be made to structure and conduct the study. Clearly and simply defining the purpose of the study also helps to avoid diffusion of activities with the attendant waste of time and money.

Determine the Type of Study Being Planned

There are many different types of research projects. It is important to define the kind of project being contemplated because the structure of the project will vary, as will the approach to conducting the study and the use of the results. Some examples of different types of studies are:

- Clinical trial
- Clinical laboratory experimentation
- Basic science
- Testing of a product for a manufacturer
- Methods development
- Case report
- Summary of data (existing or to be collected)

Chapter 1 describes the different types of study design in more detail.

Determine the Skills Needed

Laboratory Procedures

It is important to determine whether the study can be conducted using procedures already existing in the investigator's laboratory. If it is necessary to establish new procedures to carry out the research project, this adds considerably to the time and expense involved and to the complexity and uncertainty of the project. It is often easy to conceive of a project that involves a method with which the investigator is not familiar, only to discover that the reason that the project has not already been done by someone else is that the methods are more complex than anticipated or they do not exactly give the kind of data needed. This may provide a separate opportunity for publication, however. If considerable work is necessary to develop or implement a new method, this might become a separate publishable project. If so, the same planning and forethought should be applied to this "subproject" as to the overall project.

Laboratory Personnel

A parallel to examining whether the methods exist in the investigator's laboratory is whether personnel with the required skills are already part of the group that will conduct the study. While this usually does not influence publication, it is an important part of planning the project.

Clinical Expertise

If the study involves patients or data relating to the clinical care of patients, those conducting the study must have clinical expertise.

Theoretical Expertise

In addition to considering the procedures to be used and the personnel required, it is necessary to decide whether the investigator knows all the background and related information needed to successfully complete the study. If not, the type of expertise needed should be identified and a determination made as to whether it can be obtained. This could be accomplished, for instance, by the investigator studying advanced tests or learning new techniques, or by involving a collaborator who has the needed expertise. The availability of this expertise is essential in order to have a strong and successful project, and it can become a very important factor in the publication of results as well. It is likely that any journal to which the results are submitted will use individuals with considerable expertise as reviewers and if the investigators lack this expertise, the report may not withstand peer review.

Determine the Nature and Extent of the Statistical Involvement Needed

Very early in the design of a project, the type of data that will be produced should be considered and the requirements for its analysis must be determined. On this basis, the investigator can determine whether he or she has the statistical skills needed or if statistical consultation is indicated. In most major studies it is advisable to seek the advice of a biostatistician while the study is being planned. Quite often, investigators are naive about the complexities of collecting, managing, and analyzing data. No sophisticated analysis procedure can overcome the limitations of data not obtained in the proper form or under the proper conditions. Thus, if there is any question in the investigator's mind, statistical consultation should be obtained while the study design is being developed. Then the data can be obtained in the proper manner and format so that it will not only be valid but also facilitate the analysis.

Determine Whether Coinvestigators or Consultants Are Needed

On the basis of the steps described above, it is possible to decide whether all of the skills and expertise needed for the project are available in the participants already involved in the project. If not, the additional expertise must be sought. This is usually done by involving others either as coinvestigators or as consultants. It is wise to consider whether coinvestigators or consultants are likely to warrant inclusion as authors in the resulting manuscript. Planning in this regard can help to ensure their inclusion in data analysis and manuscript development, as appropriate, and to avoid subsequent controversy.

Determine Source Material Needed for the Project

Most projects require some kind of source material, and it is essential to ensure that adequate amounts of the proper material will be available for the study. Materials may range from blood samples or rare reagents to records or data elements. If the investigator does not realize that the materials are inadequate until the study begins, the study may suffer delays, cost more, or even be impossible to complete. The source of material is also important in the publication of results, because it must be possible to clearly state this source. If the materials, such as special reagents, are provided by others not involved with the study, consideration must be given to how these key materials will be obtained, their source documented, and the investigator who provided them recognized in the final report.

Prepare a Written Description of the Project

When the above steps have been completed, they should be described in writing and merged into a written plan for the study. This document will have several uses. First of all, the exercise of putting the plans down in writing often brings to light unresolved issues or gaps in the plans. As noted earlier, a description of the reason for doing the study serves as a basis for the introduction of the report of the study. An introduction also forces the investigator to describe the value of the study to convince others that the study is worthwhile. This also serves as a rationale for the funding. A detailed protocol is critical to the accurate conduct of the study and often serves as a starting point for the methods section of the resulting manuscript. In addition, an extremely valuable use of the document is to educate and build involvement in the study by the people who will be carrying out the work. It is essential that they know the purpose of the study and the reasons why the study is thought to be valuable. Sharing the written plan with them is one part of accomplishing this.

Prepare for and Obtain Human Investigation Approval

Any study involving human subjects or material obtained from human subjects must have the approval of an Institutional Review Board (IRB). Assurance that the study was approved by an IRB will be required by journals considering publishing the report of the research. The requirements for membership on, and the conduct of, an IRB are clearly defined by the Department of Health and Human Services. All major research institutions have such a board and if the investigator's organization does not, arrangements should be made to have the project reviewed by a neighboring board or by freestanding boards that will conduct such a review for a fee. This review will involve submission of a study protocol and forms to be used to obtain consent from people who are being studied or who provide material being studied. The material submitted to the IRB must describe how the subjects will be selected, whether they receive any benefit from participating in the study, methods to be used to provide confidentiality, responsibility for adverse effects on subjects in the study, and information the subjects receive about the study and their participation. These same issues must be addressed even if the study involves only blood samples from, or data about, the research subjects. Chapter 4 discusses IRBs in more detail.

Identify and Deal With Any Conflicts of Interest

Because of the increasing involvement of investigators with commercial companies and the wider variety of sources of funds supporting research, it is increasingly possible that someone conducting a study may be involved with an organization that would be affected by the outcome of the study. In general, the concern about a conflict of interest focuses on financial conflicts. For instance, if one of the investigators is a consultant to, or owns stock in, a company whose products are being studied or whose products would be affected by the results of the study, this represents a conflict of interest. This does not mean that such studies cannot be done, but thorough disclosure must be made to the funding agencies, IRBs, and when the results are prepared for presentation or publication. Most research institutions have specific procedural requirements and may require a specific separate approval of industry-sponsored projects.

Disseminating the Results

Early in the planning of the study, it is important to form a concept of what will be done with the results. Forming an idea of how the results will be used also facilitates several of the decisions described above. The results of the study may be used in many different ways, depending upon the reasons for the study and the type of study being carried out. In any case, the results of the study should be summarized in written form to document the work. The nature and extent of the summary may vary considerably depending upon the nature of the project and the reason for conducting it. For instance, in addition to the results being published, they may be used to make operational decisions after presentation to blood center management or staff, to attempt to influence the behavior of physicians or hospital staff, or to provide feedback to the organization supporting the project. It is best to have at least a general idea as to what will be done with the results before beginning the study because this will help in making specific decisions during the study. For publication, there are many options, including: peer-reviewed journals, books or monographs, workshop materials, non-peer-reviewed journals or magazines provided to professionals in that special field of work, newsletters, publications of organizations for their own use such as a company brochure, etc. Usually, the investigators have a good idea of the type of publication that should result from the project, but it is desirable to consider this early in the planning process to ensure that the project is organized in a way to provide the best possible chance of the desired publication. A full discussion of each of these options is beyond the scope of this chapter. Publication in a peer-reviewed journal is described in detail, however.

Journals

Some journals are the official journal of an organization or association. Examples of this are *Transfusion* (American Association of Blood Banks), *Blood* (American Society of Hematology), *Human Immunology* (American Society of Histocompatibility and Immunogenetics), *JAMA* (American Medical Association), *New England Journal of Medicine* (Massachusetts Medical Society), *Annals of Internal Medicine* (American College of Physicians), *Science* (American Association for the Advancement of Science), *Vox Sanguinis* (International Society of Blood Transfusion), and *Journal of Clinical Apheresis* (American Society for Apheresis). Journals that represent a particular organization may be owned by the organization or the publisher. Other journals are not associated with a particular organization and are produced by a publisher to fill a perceived need for a vehicle to make information available. Examples of this type of journal are *Transfusion Medicine Reviews*, *Plasma Therapy*, and the *American Journal of Medicine*.

For most journals, the Editor and the Associate Editors are volunteers appointed by either the organization that sponsors the journal or the publisher. In some cases, when the responsibility is for a large number of manuscripts, the organization or publisher may employ the editor as a full-time staff person. Once the Editor is appointed, that individual usually selects the Associate Editors in a way that provides a mix of expertise among the Editor and Associate Editors to cover the breadth of articles submitted to the particular journal. This usually means that the Editor and the Associate Editors are all in different institutions, and use electronic technology to communicate about manuscripts under consideration. Some journals with a very large circulation (*JAMA, New England Journal of Medicine*) maintain a paid staff of Editors housed in the journal's Editorial Office. This makes it possible for the group of Editors to have regular, frequent meetings during which final decisions are made regarding the manuscripts under consideration.

Peer-reviewed journals publish original research, meaning that the material would not have been published previously. Peer review is the cornerstone method of ensuring the quality and integrity of the journal. These journals send the manuscripts submitted for their consideration to other experts in the field and take their comments into consideration when making a decision regarding publication.

Presentation of the results of a study at a meeting from which an abstract is published does not preclude publication of the full report of the study in a peer-reviewed journal. Most journals have guidelines defining the extent to which the material can be previously published. For instance, this usually is defined as publication of an abstract or synopsis of not more than 500 words. One potential problem is that occasionally the organization or company sponsoring a meeting wishes to publish the presentations in a monograph. Usually, the material in such articles becomes sufficiently long and detailed that journals consider this to be prior publication and will not consider it as new original research when it is submitted to the journal. If authors have any doubt as to whether publication of portions of their research or presentation of material at a meeting might jeopardize later publication, the author should contact the Editor of the journal to which the manuscript will be submitted in order to obtain advice about specific situations.

Selecting a Journal

When a decision has been made to prepare a written report of a research project, some thought should be given to the journal to which the report will be submitted. The target audience should be identified; this will help in the decision. For instance, others doing similar research or individuals who would use the results of the research would read different journals than those people working in the investigator's major field. The researcher may forgo the visibility that often results from publication in a journal that would be seen by people practicing in the author's main field and choose instead a journal read by others doing similar research. In transfusion medicine, these trade-offs are illustrated by the decision whether to publish in the journal *Transfusion*, which would be seen by most people working in transfusion medicine, or a clinical journal if the report deals with the medical use of a blood component, or a basic scientific journal if the work involves biochemistry or other more basic information. The main point is that the researcher should consider the message to be delivered and the audience to whom the message is intended. Then the journal can be selected. At that point, it is probably prudent to review the situation to determine whether, on the basis of the target journal's content, it is likely the editors would be interested in the manuscript being developed.

When the desired journal has been identified, there are several steps in the submission, review, and publication process that should be considered by the report's author(s).

Instructions to Authors

Each journal publishes, usually in the January issue, instructions that authors should follow in preparing manuscripts. It is important to read these instructions carefully and develop the manuscript according to these instructions. Sending the manuscript in the proper format will facilitate the review and speed the process of publication because modifications in format will not be necessary. If the submitted manuscript differs extensively from the journal's format, the manuscript may be returned to the authors without consideration for publication. Failure to follow the journal's format suggests carelessness on the part of the investigators. The instructions to authors will describe the format to be used for the article. The format concerns the different sections of the manuscript and, generally, what each should contain. There may also be instructions about the preparation and format of the abstract. In addition, the items to be included with the manuscript will be listed. These include any consent or copyright release; signatures of coauthors; how figures should be labeled; the required number of copies of manuscript, figures, and tables; whether electronic files can be sent; and any required submission/review fee. The instructions may also mention some items of style such as the use of certain terms, abbreviations, or international units of measure.

Submitting the Manuscript

Once the manuscript has been prepared in the proper format according to the journal's instructions to authors and all of the required materials have been gathered, the material is sent to the journal. A cover letter should be written to include any specific points required by the journal. If certifications are necessary regarding authorship, conflict of interest, etc, these statements can either be included in the letter or in a separate document in the submission. Most journals require some standard wording about the author's responsibility for the material and include a copyright release. These statements are usually described in the Instructions to Authors.

Usually, the journal will require a statement regarding potential conflict of interest if the study involves commercial products. In this situation, the authors will be required to indicate whether they have a financial involvement with the manufacturer. Examples of financial involvement are owning stock, serving as a paid member of a board or advisory committee, or receiving consulting fees.

It is customary to list the sources of financial support for a study, but this is especially important for studies of commercial products. It will be necessary to indicate whether the manufacturer funded the study. This does not mean that the journal will not publish the report but it places the emphasis on disclosure. It is essential that the journal's editors, reviewers, and readers be aware if the investigators/authors received personal compensation and/or if the study was funded by the manufacturer of the product being studied.

Editorial Office

When the manuscript is received in the journal's Editorial Office, it is logged in and an initial reading is done by the Journal Editor or an Associate Editor. In some journals, this initial reading may be done by an Editorial Assistant. As noted earlier, the Associate Editors have been selected to provide a mix of expertise to cover the breadth of material usually submitted to the journal. The manuscript is then "assigned" to one of the Associate Editors who has expertise related to the content of the manuscript.

The materials submitted with the manuscript will be reviewed to determine whether all of the required documents, certifications, and related materials have been provided. If not, the author will be asked for the missing material. If there are major omissions, the manuscript may be held and the review process not begun until the missing material is provided. Thus, it is in the author's interest to review the instructions to authors carefully and be sure that all the requested materials have been included when the manuscript is submitted.

Review Process

The Associate Editor assigned to process the manuscript sends it for peer review to (usually) two individuals who are experts in the subject of the manuscript. These may be members of the journal's Editorial Board or other individuals known to the Associate Editor who is handling the particular manuscript. Usually, the journal attempts to use preferentially members of its own Editorial Board. Some general medical journals such as *JAMA* or the *New England Journal of Medicine* have a very small editorial board; thus, most of the reviews are done by invited experts.

The reviewer is provided with instructions regarding the types of issues the journal wishes the reviewer to consider and about which the journal seeks the reviewer's opinion. Examples of these types of issues include: research design, relevance of the topic, adequacy of the data, appropriateness of statistics, appropriateness of subjects or biologic material being studied, whether conclusions can be supported by the data presented, general organization of the manuscript, and appropriateness of the subject for the readers of that journal. Usually, the reviewers' comments are divided into general ones about the appropriateness of the subject, research design, or conclusions, and specific comments about certain terms, data elements, table format, organization, or statistics. While comments regarding grammar or sentence structure are helpful, the primary focus of this review should be the scientific or medical merit of the manuscript.

Because the reviewers are volunteers taking their time to provide a service to the journal and the researchers involved, the journal is not in a position to "control" the reviewers' promptness or effectiveness. Effective reviews involve a detailed critique of the material done in a thoughtful, constructive manner. Disparaging comments are neither helpful nor appropriate. In addition, brief reviews that provide only generalities are not helpful. Examples of these kinds of comments are "this is a good study that ought to be published" or "this study has little redeeming value and I cannot recommend it for publication." Journals keep track of the responsiveness and quality of reviews provided by different individuals and may stop sending manuscripts to reviewers who do not provide a timely and effective review.

Author's Revisions

Virtually every review results in some comments that are appropriate to bring to the attention of the author. Thus, almost every manuscript is returned to the author for additional work. When the reviewed manuscript is returned to the author, a cover letter from the Associate Editor will indicate the action the author is asked to take. The letter may give a fairly clear indication of the journal's interest in publishing the manuscript. These comments could range from, "We are very interested in your manuscript if you are able to revise it in accordance with the reviewers' comments," or, alternatively, "The reviewers' comments raise some very major questions about your manuscript; we are willing to continue considering your report if you can revise it to address the reviewers' concerns." Regardless of how specific the Associate Editor indicates interest in the manuscript, he or she will indicate whether the author is being asked to revise the manuscript.

If the manuscript is to be revised, the author should address each point raised by each reviewer. It is not necessary to agree with every comment from a reviewer. The author should make a decision whether to accept the reviewer's comment and make the suggested change. It is much appreciated by the Associate Editor handling the manuscript if the author in a separate cover letter lists each comment made by the reviewer and then describes either the change that has been made in the manuscript or the reason for disagreeing with the reviewer's comment and not implementing the change. The revisions should be made as promptly as possible. Most journals have a maximal period during which they will hold the manuscript file open and continue to process revisions of the original manuscript. After that time, the manuscript would be treated as a new submission requiring an additional submission fee and a new review process.

Re-Review

When the revised manuscript is received, the Associate Editor will review the original reviewers' comments and Associate Editor's notes. If extensive revision was required or if fundamental questions were raised such as the structure of the study, the conclusions reached, or extrapolations of the results, the manuscript will probably be sent out for re-review. Re-review is usually done by the original reviewers. This will extend the time required for a publication decision to be reached. If no fundamental issues were raised in the original review and if the original comments were fairly straightforward, the Associate Editor may elect to reread the manuscript and the author's explanation of the revision and make a decision regarding publication. The Associate Editor will usually make a decision on the manuscript within a few days or a couple of weeks, thus shortening the manuscript processing time.

If the manuscript is subjected to re-review, the Associate Editor will usually be careful to limit the re-review comments to the issues raised by the initial review. Of course, if a new substantive issue is raised because the revision has changed the content of the report, this will be addressed. Also, if an important issue was overlooked in the initial review, this must be addressed. However, the Associate Editor must be careful not to be drawn into a sequence of finding a new point to criticize with each revision and, thus, seem to be changing the expectations with each review step.

Final Decision

For most journals, each Associate Editor is empowered to make the decision regarding publication. The Associate Editor may consult with the Journal Editor before making a decision, but that is the Associate Editor's option. A "quality assurance" system is usually used by which the Journal Editor reviews the rejected manuscripts to ensure that the Associate Editors' decision-making is consistent with the standards that the Journal Editor wishes to maintain for the journal. Other journals, usually only large ones with a paid full-time staff, have frequent and regular meetings of the Associate Editors and the Journal Editor at which the final decisions are made regarding publication. This is also done by a few journals, where all editors are at the same institution.

When a decision regarding publication has been made, the author will be notified promptly. If the manuscript is accepted, the letter will contain specific instructions as to what, if anything, the author should do next. Usually, nothing is required until the proofs are available for review.

If the manuscript is not accepted, the letter may explain the reasons rather specifically or it may be somewhat vague. It is most helpful to the author if the letter can be rather specific, and most journals try to do this. However, sometimes there are no specific "criticisms" of the manuscript, but it may not be considered of enough interest for the journal's audience, or the general quality of the report may not be strong enough to warrant acceptance. In this case, the letter usually is more general, saying that the journal receives many manuscripts and this particular one is not strong enough to be accepted.

Production

During the production process, the manuscript is copyedited; typeset page proofs are printed; the sequence of articles is determined; advertising pages are inserted; page numbers are assigned; and the issue is printed, bound, and mailed.

Editing

Once a manuscript has been accepted for publication, it is reviewed by a Copy Editor. The purpose of this editing process is to ensure grammatical correctness and to apply the journal's particular style to the manuscript. Style choices refer to the use of certain standard terms or abbreviations, decisions as to when the active and passive voice will be used, the manner in which tables are formatted, how figure legends are used, etc. There is considerable standardization of terminology and abbreviations of words and terms commonly used by each particular journal. In addition, most Journal Editors prefer that their journal articles have a rather consistent sentence style.

There is some variation, however, in the degree to which different journals apply their own styles. Some journals prefer that every manuscript flow and read in a more standard, consistent manner, whereas other journals are willing to accept articles with considerably more variability in the way they read, giving a more heterogeneous feel to the journal.

Galley or Page Proof Review

Printed proofs of the manuscript will be sent to the primary author for review. Careful review is important because this is the author's last chance to correct any specific errors, not only in grammar or spelling, but also in figures or numbers in tables. Because proofs are generated rather far along in the production process, prompt review of the proofs and their return to the publisher are important in order for the journal to maintain its production schedule. The Copy Editor may have questions to which the author is asked to respond. These will be noted on the proofs and the author can respond by writing the answer on the proofs. If the author has questions or concerns, these should be brought to the attention of the Copy Editor either by making a note on the proofs or by contacting the Editorial Office.

Publication

The printing, assembly, and mailing of the journal may be done in or near the publisher's facility or in a remote location. Journals may be mailed by first class or other classes of mail, so receipt by the reader may be at different intervals from the publication date, depending on the class of mail used and the location of the recipient.

Reprints

When the journal prints the issue containing the manuscript, it is possible to produce at a fairly low cost individual reprints of each article. These are usually made available to the authors at a modest charge. In the past, it was customary as a courtesy for the author to provide these reprints to other researchers who would write to request copies of the article. This practice continues and most authors order reprints of their articles. However, the practice has declined in recent years with the decreasing availability of funds.

Reprints should be ordered at the time the final proofs are returned to the publisher. Usually, reprint request forms will be included with these proofs. While it may be possible to obtain reprints later, this may be more costly because the publisher must retrieve the original files, select the single article from the issue, and run the press in a less than cost-effective manner. Also, with modern desk-to-plate technology, there are no negatives and the plates are recycled; a publisher may not be able to produce reprints of the article after a certain period, which will vary with different publishers.

Conclusions

The major function of journals is to assist authors and researchers to disseminate the results of their work. Conducting a research project, analyzing the data, preparing a written report, submitting it to a journal, and going through the process of publication takes time, perseverance, and hard work. The result should be the publication of an attractive article that effectively communicates the work and the author's views about its significance, all of which should provide a sense of gratification to the author when the issue containing the article is received.

In: Brecher ME, Busch MP, eds.
Research Design and Analysis
Bethesda, MD: American Association of Blood Banks, 1998

6

NHLBI Support for Biomedical Research and Training

George J. Nemo, PhD

THE NATIONAL HEART, LUNG, and Blood Institute (NHLBI) supports a national program of research, research training, and career development in diseases of the heart, blood vessels, lung, and blood; blood resources; and sleep disorders. This chapter provides an overview of the Institute's biomedical research and training programs, the process of developing Institute-initiated research activities, the Division of Blood Diseases and Resources Program in Blood Resources and Transfusion Medicine, and funding mechanisms available to the scientific community.

Program Overview

The NHLBI is part of the National Institutes of Health (NIH). The NHLBI was established in 1948 as the National Heart Institute with a mission to support research and training in the prevention, treatment, and diagnosis of cardiovascular diseases. Twenty-four years later, through the National Heart, Blood Vessel, Lung, and Blood Act (P.L. 92-423), Congress mandated the Institute to expand and coordinate its activities in an accelerated attack against heart, blood vessel, lung,

---

George J. Nemo, PhD, Group Leader, Transfusion Medicine Scientific Research Group, Division of Blood Diseases and Resources, National Heart, Lung, and Blood Institute, Bethesda, Maryland

and blood diseases. The renamed National Heart, Lung, and Blood Institute expanded its scientific areas of interest and intensified its efforts related to research on all diseases under its purview.

The mission of the NHLBI is to provide leadership for a national program in the diseases identified in the expanded legislation and in blood resources and sleep disorders. The Institute supports a coordinated program of basic research, clinical investigations and trials, observational studies, and demonstration and education activities in its own laboratories (intramural) and by scientific institutions and individuals supported by research grants and contracts (extramural). It supports research training and career development of new and established researchers in the fundamental sciences and clinical disciplines to enable them to conduct research related to the mission of the Institute through individual and institutional research training awards and career development awards. The Institute conducts educational activities including development and dissemination of materials for health professionals and the public with emphasis on prevention.

The NHLBI program is implemented through five extramural units: the Division of Heart and Vascular Diseases, the Division of Lung Diseases, the Division of Blood Diseases and Resources, the Division of Epidemiology and Clinical Applications, and the National Center on Sleep Disorders Research. There is also one intramural unit, the Division of Intramural Research. The Divisions and the Center pursue their own scientific mission but cooperate in areas of shared interest such as prevention, education, and control.

Management of extramural research and training activities in hematology resides in the Division of Blood Diseases and Resources. The Division develops and administers programs to reduce morbidity and mortality caused by blood diseases and to lead to their primary prevention. Diseases addressed include hemophilia, Cooley's anemia, sickle cell disease, and disorders of hemostasis and thrombosis. The Division also has a major responsibility to ensure the safety and adequacy of the nation's blood supply. A full range of activities, including studies of transmission of infectious disease through transfusion, development of methods to inactivate infectious agents in donated blood, improvement of blood donor screening procedures, research to reduce human error in transfusion medicine, and studies of emerging infectious agents that may be transmitted by blood transfusion, is being performed to achieve this goal.

Dissemination of research findings to the medical community through workshops, conferences, and consensus development conferences is an important function of the Division. Efforts to disseminate research results have been conducted in such topics as plasma transfusion, platelet transfusion therapy, diagnosis of deep-vein thrombosis, impact of routine human immunodeficiency virus (HIV) antibody testing of blood and plasma donors on public health, stem cell therapy, immune function in sickle cell disease, and management of patients with hepatitis C virus (HCV).

To meet its overall responsibilities, the Division maintains a program of grants, contracts, training and career development awards, and academic awards. Specialized Centers of Research (SCOR) in thrombosis, transfusion biology and medicine, and hematopoietic stem cell biology, and Comprehensive Centers in sickle cell disease are being supported.

The Division of Blood Diseases and Resources is organized into two major program areas, the Blood Diseases Program and the Blood Resources Program. The Blood Diseases Program is subdivided into two scientific research groups: cellular hematology and sickle cell disease. The Blood Resources Program consists of three scientific research groups: bone marrow transplantation, transfusion medicine, and thrombosis and hemostasis.

Investigator-Initiated Research

Approximately 68% of NHLBI's fiscal year 1997 total extramural funds supported individual research projects conceived and conducted by scientists based at universities, nonprofit research foundations, and private research laboratories. Support is generally provided through research project grants dealing with all phases of medical research, from molecular and cellular investigations to studies of new drugs to treat human disease. In fiscal year 1997, the NHLBI funded 821 competing research project grants; the most common type, known as an R01 grant, supports a single project and a single principal investigator. Some research project grants are program project grants, which support multidisciplinary projects conducted by several investigators working on different aspects of a research problem.

Institute-Initiated Research Programs: The Process of Planning, Developing, and Implementing Initiatives

Approximately 28% of the Institute's total extramural budget in fiscal year 1997 supported research that was initiated by the Institute. There is an ongoing process within the Institute to evaluate broad areas of science and identify areas of research where special emphasis is warranted. If, for example, the Institute is convinced that a particular area of science offers opportunity, but extramural scientists are not generating research proposals in that area, the Institute may decide to organize a workshop or conference to identify specific scientific needs and opportunities, stimulate research applications, and attract scientists into the field. Or, if the Institute wants to encourage extramural scientists to apply their particular skills to a new challenge, the Institute may generate an initiative and formally solicit research grant applications or contract proposals from the scientific community. Each NHLBI initiative represents the outcome of numerous discussions and reviews by representatives of the scientific community and by Institute advisory groups and special emphasis panels. The groups and panels, together with professional societies and NHLBI staff, continually review the progress of research in the NHLBI program areas and identify research topics that are worth pursuing. On the advice and recommendations of the various groups, Division staff members develop the highest priority areas into proposed initiatives.

An initiative must compete in importance and for funds not only with other initiatives but also with other Institute programs, including investigator-initiated research. Goals for initiatives can be of different types. Examples include bringing new scientists, new disciplines, new approaches, and adequate resources to promising but relatively little-studied areas; accelerating activity and capitalizing upon an opportunity in an especially important area; establishing a collaborative approach to a problem; or announcing specific needs of the Institute. Some initiatives support other Institute activities, for example, providing animal resources or fabricating devices, assessing a target population through a survey, or developing a specific test methodology. Occasionally, an initiative is required to carry out a congressionally mandated activity.

Initiatives are first evaluated by the Division with regard to scientific merit, timeliness, feasibility, and cost. Initiatives that satisfy these criteria are then presented to the Institute Director for discussion and review.

To provide maximum flexibility to the Institute in implementing research initiatives, the National Heart, Lung, and Blood Advisory Council considers initiatives at each of its meetings. The initiatives are presented at the Advisory Council meeting during open session. Council comments are solicited for each initiative, and Council advice on special areas of emphasis is encouraged.

Council comments are considered further by NHLBI staff and, on occasion, by other advisors to determine the appropriate course of action. When an initiative has been reviewed by the Council, it is considered for issuance by the NHLBI Director. Initiatives may or may not be approved for release, depending upon several factors such as review workloads, program priorities, the proposed funding mechanism and the Institute budget. When the Director approves an initiative for release, the responsible NHLBI staff member(s) develops the solicitation document, which is reviewed and must be approved by the NHLBI and the NIH. An announcement of availability of the solicitation is released in the *NIH Guide to Grants and Contracts.*

Solicitations are generally released as either Request for Applications (RFAs) for grants or for cooperative agreements, or Request for Proposals (RFPs) for contracts. For each of the solicitations, the Institute outlines goals, approaches, and other requirements in detail; announces the availability of resources and their approximate magnitude; sets a single due date for the responses; and maintains a coordinating or collaborative role with the program participants. Applications are reviewed under the auspices of the Institute's Division of Extramural Affairs by a specially convened expert group. The results of the review are considered by Institute staff in terms of scientific and program balance as well as available resources. A program plan is prepared that documents these results. For grants and cooperative agreements, the plan undergoes Council review. For contracts, a series of programmatic and administrative reviews is conducted according to the Federal Acquisition Regulations. Once the awards are made, NHLBI staff arrange periodic meetings of the specific program investigators and other relevant NHLBI investigators to foster communication and exchange scientific information during the course of the program.

Another approach for stimulating research is the program announcement (PA). In contrast to the RFA and RFP mechanisms, a PA indicates a special interest of the Institute in supporting an activity or in reaching a goal, but it neither details the goals or approaches nor establishes requirements. No special resources are available and no single due date for applications is specified. Applications submitted in response to a PA receive the same study section review under the auspices of the Center for Scientific Review as other investigator-initiated grant applications, but following study section review, the Institute's programmatic interests enter into their further assessment. After the awards are made, there is ordinarily no coordinating or collaborative role by Institute staff other than the regular administration of research grants.

Applications and proposals submitted in response to RFAs and RFPs compete among themselves for specific "set-aside" funds. Applications submitted in response to PAs compete with other investigator-initiated applications for funding.

Distribution of the Division of Blood Diseases and Resources Budget by Funding Mechanism

The Division of Blood Diseases and Resources budget in fiscal year 1997 totaled about $242 million. Investigator-initiated awards consisting primarily of individual research project grants (R01s) and program project grants (P01s) received approximately 61% of the funding (Fig 6-1). Conversely, Institute-initiated research activities consisting of RFAs, Centers, and contracts accounted for about 33% of the

NHLBI RESEARCH AND TRAINING SUPPORT 155

	Funds*	%
Investigator Inititated Research	148,666	61.5
RFA	28,044	11.6
Training (NRSA)	7,624	3.2
Centers	32,448	13.4
Research Career (K)	6,022	2.5
Contracts	18,935	7.8
Totals	241,739	100.0

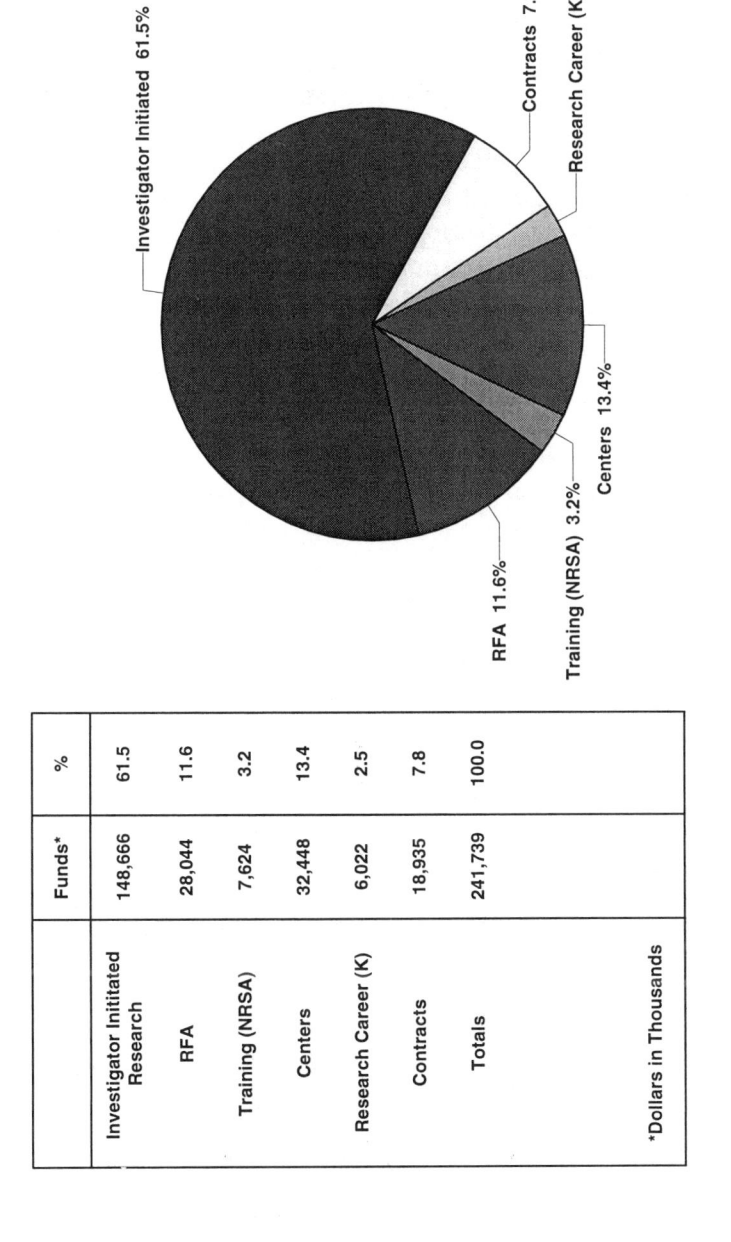

*Dollars in Thousands

Figure 6-1. Division of Blood Diseases and Resources—distribution of budget by funding mechanisms for fiscal year 1997.

Division budget. Approximately 11% of the budget supported R01 grant applications solicited by the RFA mechanism. Centers, which include Sickle Cell Disease Centers and SCORs in transfusion biology and medicine, thrombosis, and hematopoietic stem cell biology, account for about 13% of the Division budget. Contracts utilize about 8% and research training and career development programs totaled about 6%.

An analysis of the budget in the Blood Resources Program reveals major differences in the use of funding mechanisms by the three scientific research groups (Table 6-1). Most of the funds in the Thrombosis and Hemostasis Scientific Research Group, about 83%, supported investigator-initiated research activities. In contrast, 42% of funds in the Transfusion Medicine Scientific Research Group and about 30% of funds in the Bone Marrow Transplantation Scientific Research Group supported investigator-initiated research.

Table 6-1. Blood Resources Program—Distribution of Funds* in Fiscal Year 1997

	Thrombosis and Hemostasis		Transfusion Medicine		Bone Marrow Transplantation	
	Funds	%	Funds	%	Funds	%
Investigator-Initiated Research	77,679	82.8	15,901	42.0	3,543	29.6
RFA	5,838	6.2	6,182	16.3	0	0.0
Training (NRSA)	3,263	3.5	675	1.8	872	7.3
Centers	4,136	4.4	3,969	10.5	0	0.0
Research Career	2,929	3.1	52	0.1	331	2.8
Contracts	0	0.0	11,046	29.2	7,212	60.3
Totals	93,845	100.0	37,825	100.0	11,958	100.0

*Dollars in thousands
RFA = request for application; NRSA = National Research Service Award

Institute-initiated research consisting of RFAs, Centers and contracts received approximately 60% of funds in the Bone Marrow Transplantation Scientific Research Group and 56% in the Transfusion Medicine Scientific Research Group. Only about 11% of funds in the Thrombosis and Hemostasis Scientific Research Group were devoted to Institute-initiated activities. Hence, most of the budget of the Thrombosis and Hemostasis Scientific Research Group provides support to investigators who initiate their own research projects. The majority of funds in the Transfusion Medicine and Bone Marrow Transplantation Scientific Research Groups, however, support extramural programs initiated by the Institute.

Transfusion Medicine Scientific Research Group: Current Institute-Initiated Research Activities

Descriptions of active Institute-initiated research projects in the transfusion medicine program are presented below according to types of solicitation and funding mechanism.

Request for Applications: Grants

SCOR in Transfusion Biology and Medicine

The objectives of the SCOR program in Transfusion Biology and Medicine are to improve the safety and efficacy of blood and blood components, define the indications for their use, evaluate and possibly modify immunologic responsiveness following their administration, and develop and evaluate alternative treatment strategies that substitute for certain of their functions or stimulate their endogenous production so as to reduce transfusion needs. This initiative also encourages the use of new and innovative technologies to pursue fundamental research studies in transfusion biology and clinical investigations in transfusion medicine. The goals of this program are to understand better the basic biology of transfusion; make optimal use of blood, blood components, and plasma protein derivatives in specific replacement therapy; and improve transfusion practice.

Trial to Reduce Alloimmunization to Platelets (TRAP)

This is a multi-institutional, randomized, blinded trial to determine if procedures to remove or alter leukocytes in platelet preparations either by filtration or treatment with ultraviolet B (UV-B) irradiation would prevent platelet alloantibodies and refractoriness to platelet transfusions in patients undergoing marrow ablative chemotherapy for acute myelogenous leukemia (AML). The main manuscript from TRAP was published recently documenting the value of leukocyte reduction by filtration and UV-B irradiation of platelet preparations in preventing alloimmune platelet refractoriness and alloimmunization in patients with AML. Trial investigators are currently preparing secondary manuscripts.

Hemoglobin-Based Oxygen Carriers: Mechanisms of Toxicity

The objective of this program is to obtain an understanding of the mechanisms of toxicity of hemoglobin-based oxygen carriers. This program is addressing a variety of fundamental questions including: 1) What are the mechanisms of vasoactivity of hemoglobin solutions? 2) How do protein modifications affect vasoactivity? 3) What mechanisms are involved in stimulation of inflammation mediators by hemoglobin-based oxygen carriers? 4) What animal or in-vitro models are best to study toxic effects of oxygen carriers? and 5) What are the long-term (metabolic and pharmacologic) effects of oxygen carriers?

In-Vitro Inactivation of Transfusion-Transmitted Viruses in Cellular Blood Components

The purpose of this program is to develop simple, cost-effective inactivation procedures to destroy the infectivity of transfusion-transmitted viruses in blood and blood components while maintaining the therapeutic effectiveness of the components.

Human HIV Monoclonal Antibodies in Immunotherapy

The objectives of this program are to develop broadly neutralizing human HIV monoclonal antibodies (MoAbs), develop animal model systems to evaluate their effectiveness as passive immunotherapy for prevention and treatment of HIV infection, and establish an efficient in-vitro neutralization test (or other assay system) for validation of the animal studies. The goal of this program is to produce sufficient effective MoAbs (or mixtures of MoAbs), perhaps in combination with other products, and make them available to examine the efficacy of newly developed products in clinical trials.

Viability and Function of Transfused Platelets

The purpose of this program is to conduct studies on the alterations produced in blood platelets during collection, processing, and storage; on the development of detection techniques for monitoring viability and function of platelets after collection and processing, and during storage; and on the prevention of defects responsible for loss of function. The goal of this initiative is to improve the viability and function of transfused platelets.

Request for Proposals: Contracts

Retrovirus Epidemiology Donor Study (REDS)

This multicenter program was established to determine accurately the incidence and prevalence of retrovirus markers in blood donors; to evaluate the demographic, risk factor, and behavioral characteristics of blood donors; to establish blood specimen repositories; to evaluate new tests for known viruses; and to serve as a sentinel for as-yet-unrecognized blood-borne viruses that pose a risk to the safety of the blood supply.

Natural History of Posttransfusion Hepatitis

The objective of this multicenter study is to obtain clinical, biochemical, and histological information on patients who developed HCV posttransfusion hepatitis and compare it with transfusion recipients who did not develop posttransfusion hepatitis. In this study, patients were identified who developed posttransfusion hepatitis in previously completed prospective studies and are being followed to determine the long-term consequences (morbidity and mortality) of HCV posttransfusion hepatitis.

Refinement of New Assays for Direct Detection of Viral Nucleic Acids in Donors of Blood for Transfusion and of Organs for Transplantation

This program is refining, for use in clinical laboratories, nucleic acid-based amplification techniques for the direct detection of blood-borne viruses (HIV and HCV) in individual donors of blood for transfusion and of organs for transplantation. The purpose of the new techniques is to reduce to the shortest possible time the antibody-negative window—the period of time between initial infectivity of an infectious agent and its earliest detection.

Anti-HIV Immunoglobulin in Prevention of Maternal-Fetal HIV Transmission

The objective of this multi-institutional study is to determine if HIV hyperimmune globulin (HIVIG) given to HIV-positive pregnant women during the second and third trimester of pregnancy reduces the likelihood of maternal-fetal HIV transmission. Patient recruitment was terminated last year because the HIV transmission rate was too low to provide sufficient power to distinguish between the two arms of the study. Patients and controls previously entered into the trial continue to be evaluated prospectively.

Virus Activation Transfusion Study (VATS)

This multicenter trial is designed to determine if activation of HIV and cytomegalovirus occurs following blood transfusion in HIV-infected persons, thereby adversely affecting their prognosis. This study will also evaluate the role of donor leukocytes producing this activation by examining the effect of removing leukocytes by filtration.

Cord Blood Stem Cell Transplantation Study (COBLT)

This multicenter study is designed to show whether umbilical cord blood stem cell transplants from unrelated, newborn donors are a safe and effective alternative to marrow transplantation for children and adults with a variety of cancers, blood diseases, and genetic disorders. The study includes a coordinating center, six transplant centers, and three cord blood collection and storage centers. This program is managed jointly by the Transfusion Medicine and Bone Marrow Transplantation Scientific Research Groups.

Maintenance of Chimpanzees for Hepatitis and AIDS Research

The Institute supports a colony of 51 chimpanzees by providing housing and veterinary medical support. These chimpanzees are available to members of the scientific community for use in experimental studies of viral hepatitis or HIV.

Maintenance of a Biological Specimen Repository

The purposes of this repository are to maintain collections of biological specimens from NHLBI-sponsored studies and, under Institute direction, to make appropriate specimens available to the scientific community for use in research related to transfusion-transmitted diseases and disorders of the blood, cardiovascular, and respiratory systems. Examples of research protocols include evaluation of more sensitive tests to detect HIV in blood donors; evaluation of newly identified agents in donated blood; study of hemostatic changes during and immediately after myocardial infarction; evaluation of hemostatic differences between patients whose vessels remain patent after thrombolytic therapy and those who suffer reclosure; and etiology of thrombotic thrombocytopenic purpura.

Types of Grant Mechanisms

The NHLBI employs a wide array of extramural funding mechanisms to fulfill its mission. The following are descriptions of some of the more common types of grant mechanisms available through the Institute.
- *Research Project Grant (R01):* Supports discrete and specific projects to be performed by one or several investigators in areas of the investigator's particular interests and competencies. The individual research project grant, commonly referred to as an R01, is considered by the biomedical research community to be the mainstay of biomedical

research. It is the standard by which research is supported and judged. Most investigator-initiated research supported by the NHLBI is provided through this mechanism.
- *Research Project (Cooperative Agreement) (U01):* Supports discrete, circumscribed projects in areas of an investigator's specific interest and competency involving substantial programmatic participation by the NHLBI during performance of the activity. The TRAP is an example of a Cooperative Agreement grant program. It was established using an RFA to solicit applications for the trial coordinating center and another RFA for clinical centers.
- *Research Program Project (P01):* Supports broadly based, multidisciplinary research projects that have specific major objectives or basic themes directed toward a well-defined research program goal. An organized group of researchers conducts individual subprojects, the results of which serve to achieve the objectives of the program project. To stabilize the base funding of P01s, the Institute has set aside a percentage of its research project grant budget for this purpose.
- *Small Research Grant (R03):* Provides limited support for extended analyses of research data generated by clinical trials, population research, and demonstration and education studies. The NHLBI instituted this program to allow investigators the opportunity to analyze existing databases for outcomes not contemplated in the original design of a study or trial. According to NHLBI policy, this award may not be used to supplement projects supported by federal or nonfederal funds, to provide interim support for projects under review by the Public Health Service, to provide support for dissertation research, to substitute for a competing renewal application, or to support pilot or feasibility studies.
- *Academic Research Enhancement Award (AREA) (R15):* Supports small-scale research projects conducted by faculty in primarily baccalaureate degree-granting domestic institutions. Grant awards are for up to $75,000 for direct costs (plus applicable indirect costs) for periods not to exceed 36 months.
- *Method to Extend Research in Time (MERIT) Award (R37):* Provides long-term research grant support to investigators whose research competency and productivity are distinctly superior

and who are likely to continue to perform in an outstanding manner. Investigators may not apply for a MERIT award; instead, they are selected by the NHLBI based on their current grant applications and their present and past grant support.
- *Small Business Technology Transfer (STTR) Grant—Phase I (R41):* Supports cooperative research and development projects between small business concerns and research institutions to establish the technical merit and feasibility of ideas that have potential for commercialization. Awards are made to small business concerns only. At least 40% of the research project is to be conducted by the small business concern and at least 30% of the work is to be conducted by the single, "partnering" research institution. Support of up to $100,000 is provided for 1 year.
- *Small Business Technology Transfer (STTR) Grant—Phase II (R42):* Supports in-depth development of cooperative research and development projects between small business concerns and research institutions whose feasibility has been established in Phase I and that have potential commercialization. Awards are made to small business concerns only. A total of up to $500,000 in support is provided for 2 years.
- *Small Business Innovation Research (SBIR) Grant—Phase I (R43):* Supports projects to establish the technical merit and feasibility of research and development ideas that may ultimately lead to commercial products or services. Innovation and the potential for commercialization are among the important factors included in the review criteria used in the scientific and technical merit evaluation process. Support of up to $100,000 is provided for 6 months.
- *Small Business Innovation Research (SBIR) Grant—Phase II (R44):* Supports research project ideas that have been shown to be feasible in Phase I and that are likely to result in commercially marketable products or services. Total support of up to $750,000 is provided for 2 years.
- *Conference Grant (R13):* Provides funding for national or international conferences to coordinate and disseminate information related to program interests.
- *Demonstration and Education Research Grant (R18):* Supports studies designed to develop, test, and evaluate the ef-

fectiveness of interventions to promote health or prevent disease in defined populations.
- *Minority Investigator Research Supplements:* Provide supplemental funds to ongoing R01, R15, R18, R37, P01, or U01 research grants supported by the NHLBI to recruit minority investigators to research careers in the sciences related to heart, lung, and blood diseases; blood resources; and sleep disorders.

Change in Policy Regarding Support of New Investigators

The NIH is no longer accepting grant applications for R29 (First Independent Research Support and Transition) awards. These awards, also known as FIRST awards, were designed to provide a sufficient initial period of research support for newly independent biomedical investigators to develop their research capabilities and demonstrate the merit of their research ideas. The FIRST award provided a 5-year period of research support.

Since 1986, a significant number of investigators have applied for R29 support, although most new investigators applied for R01 funding. R29 applicants have had a somewhat better award rate than new applicants for R01s. However, when subsequently applying for renewal R01 funding, applicants who received R29 funding as their initial method of support are less successful than new applicants who received an R01.

NIH's new policy was adopted after an analysis by the Working Group on New Investigators. The Working Group concluded that while new investigators applying for either R01 or R29 funding are similar, they are subject to an artificial division of applicants that leads them to grant support mechanisms, either the R01 or R29, with several differences. These differences include review criteria, requirement for letters of support, dollar and time limitations, and percentage of time required for the new investigators. Some of these differences can penalize the R29 applicant; the most significant is the dollar limitation of the R29, which is $350,000 over a 5-year period, with no single year exceeding $100,000. By having all new investigators meet the same R01 requirements, NIH will eliminate these differences. There is no set time limit, proportion of salary, or dollar cap attached to R01 grants. Letters of support are not needed. To ensure a fair scientific peer review process, NIH staff is fully explaining this change in policy to study sections and Institute Advisory Councils and establishing procedures and application forms to ensure that reviewers can clearly identify those applications that are submitted by new investigators.

Research Centers

As noted earlier, the NHLBI supports the work of SCORs and comprehensive centers.
- *Specialized Centers of Research Grant (P50):* Supports basic and clinical research related to an Institute-identified theme. The spectrum of SCOR activities comprises multidisciplinary approaches to specific disease entities or biomedical areas where research opportunities exist. The SCOR grants differ from research program project grants in that they are in response to an RFA of programmatic needs of the Institute. Centers may be asked to perform additional studies because of urgently needed information or may serve as a regional or national resource for special research needs.
- *Comprehensive Centers Grant (P60):* Supports a multipurpose unit designed to bring together into a common focus divergent but related facilities within a given community; to foster biomedical research and development at both the fundamental and clinical levels; to initiate and expand community education, screening, and counseling programs; and to educate medical and allied health professionals concerning problems of diagnosis and treatment of specific diseases such as sickle cell anemia.

Grants to Support Research Career Development

In an effort to increase and improve its support of patient-oriented research training, the NHLBI has established the following three new career development awards for patient-oriented research.
- *Mentored Patient-Oriented Research Career Development Award (K23):* This is a new mechanism to support the ca-

reer development of investigators who have made a commitment to focus their research endeavors on patient-oriented research. This mechanism provides support for up to 5 years of supervised study and research for candidates holding clinical degrees who have the potential to develop into productive, clinical investigators focusing on patient-oriented research. Salary is provided to a maximum of $75,000, with at least 75% effort being devoted to the goals of this award. Research development support may be requested for up to $25,000 per year. This award is not renewable.

- *Mid-Career Investigator Award in Patient-Oriented Research (K24):* This new mechanism provides support for outstanding clinical scientists who are within 15 years of their specialty training to allow them protected time to engage in patient-oriented research and to act as mentors for beginning clinical investigators. The NIH will provide a salary of up to $62,500 per year for 25-50% effort. Research development support may be requested for up to $25,000 per year. This award is for a maximum of 5 years. It is also renewable for an additional 5-year period if the awardee still meets the requirements.

- *Clinical Research Curriculum Award (K30):* This is a new institutional award intended to support the development of new didactic programs in clinical research at institutions that do not currently offer such programs, or to institutions with existing didactic programs to expand their programs or to improve the quality of instruction. The goal of this program is to improve the training of the participants, so that upon completion of their training, they can more effectively compete for research funding. Salary of the program director must not exceed an annual level of $125,000 plus fringe benefits (a maximum of $62,000 for 50% effort). The program director must devote at least 25% effort but no greater than 50% effort to the award. An institution may have only one K30. The award is renewable for additional 5-year periods.

In addition to these three new awards, the NHLBI also offers the Independent Scientist Award (K02) and the Mentored Clinical Scientist Development Award (K08).

- *Independent Scientist Award (K02):* The goal of this award is to enhance the research capability of promising individuals in the formative stages of their careers of independent research by freeing them from teaching, administrative, or committee responsibilities, allowing them to focus on their research project(s). This award provides support for newly independent scientists who can demonstrate the need for a period of intensive research as a means of advancing their research careers. This award provides salary only, and the applicant must have ongoing peer-reviewed research support. Salary is provided up to $50,000 per year plus fringe benefits with 75% effort. Research support may be requested for up to $15,000 per year.

- *Mentored Clinical Scientist Development Award (K08):* The objective of this award is to support the development of outstanding clinical research scientists. This mechanism provides specialized study for clinically trained professionals who are committed to a career in research and have the potential to develop into independent investigators. This supervised research experience may integrate didactic studies with laboratory or clinical research. The proposed research should have both intrinsic research importance and be a suitable vehicle for learning the methodology, theories, and conceptualizations necessary for a well-trained independent researcher. Salary is up to $50,000 per year plus fringe benefits with 75% effort. Research support may be requested up to $15,000 per year.

National Research Service Awards (NRSA)

Individual and Institutional awards provide support for individuals at various levels of career development who wish to gain additional experience in biomedical research.

- *NRSA Individual Fellowship Award (F32):* This award provides postdoctoral research training to individuals to broaden their scientific background and extend their potential for research in areas related to heart, lung, and blood diseases; blood resources; and sleep disorders. Postdoctoral fellowships are awarded for a period of 2-3 years to individuals having an appropriate sponsor and institution. The stipend is $21,000-$33,012 per year based on years of relevant postdoctoral experience. An institutional allowance of $4,000 is provided to defray fellowship expenses.

- *NRSA for Senior Fellows (F33):* This award provides experienced scientists who have at least 7 years of relevant postdoctoral research or professional experience an opportunity to make major changes in the direction of their research careers, to acquire new research capabilities, to enlarge their command of an allied research field, or to take time from regular professional responsibilities for the purpose of broadening their research capabilities in order to conduct biomedical or behavioral research. Fellowships are awarded to individuals who have an appropriate sponsor and institution. Stipends may be negotiated up to $33,012 per year with supplementation from nonfederal funds permitted. An institutional allowance of $4,000 is provided to defray fellowship expenses.
- *NRSA Institutional Research Training Award (T32):* Awards for up to 5 years are made to institutions on behalf of a training program director for pre- and postdoctoral training in areas related to heart, lung, and blood diseases; blood resources; and sleep disorders. Trainees are selected through local review established by the training program director. The stipend is $21,000 - $33,012 per year based on years of relevant postdoctoral experience. The stipend is $11,748 per year for predoctoral (MD or PhD) trainees. Support may be requested for tuition, fees, health insurance, and travel. The research training period for each trainee must be at least 2 years; postdoctoral support is limited to a maximum of 3 years. Predoctoral (MD) support for 1 year during leave from medical training is also allowed. Training-related expenses of $2,500 per postdoctoral and $1,500 per predoctoral trainee may be requested.

Minority Programs

The NHLBI supports several programs intended to encourage minority participation in research training for careers in biomedical research.
- *NRSA Predoctoral Fellowship Award for Minority Students (F31):* This is an award for well-qualified students from minority groups that are under represented in the biomedical and behavioral sciences in the United States. The fellowship provides for up to 5 years of support for research train-

ing leading to a PhD, combined MD/PhD, or other combined professional degrees in the biomedical or behavioral sciences. A stipend of $11,748 per year and an institutional allowance of $2,000 are provided. Tuition and fees will be provided in accordance with NIH policy.
- *NRSA Short-Term Training for Minority Students (T35M):* This is an institutional award for domestic nonprofit institutions or organizations engaged in health-related research to provide minority undergraduate students, graduate students, and students in health professional schools exposure to opportunities in research careers in areas relevant to heart, lung, and blood diseases; blood resources; and sleep disorders. Trainees must have completed at least one undergraduate year at an accredited school or university. The training period is 8-12 weeks at 100% effort. Stipend support for trainees is $979 per month and may be supplemented from nonfederal funds. Training and travel-related costs may be requested.
- *Minority Institution Faculty-Mentored Research Scientist Development Award (K01):* This program provides research support to faculty members at minority institutions who have the interest and potential to conduct high-quality research in the areas of heart, lung, and blood diseases, blood resources, and sleep disorders. Important goals are to enhance the institution's science programs and to assist in the acquisition of "hands on" research opportunities for minority students at the applicant's institution. Awards are for 5 years. This program is open to candidates having faculty appointments and holding PhD, MD, DVM, DO, or an equivalent professional degree. The applicant must arrange to work with an accomplished investigator at a nearby research center.
- *Mentored Research Scientist Development Award for Minority Faculty (K01):* This program provides support to underrepresented minority faculty members with varying levels of research experience to prepare them for research careers as independent investigators. The research development programs proposed for the applicant should be based on scholastic background, previous research experience, past achievements, and potential to develop into an independent investigator. The objective of the award is to develop highly trained underrepresented minority investigators

whose basic or clinical research interests are grounded in the advanced methods and experimental approaches needed to solve problems related to heart, lung, and blood diseases; blood resources; and sleep disorders.

Summary

The NHLBI supports research (investigator-initiated as well as Institute-initiated), training, and career development. One of the five distinct program units, the Division of Blood Diseases and Resources supports a full range of grants, contracts, and awards, in addition to collaborative efforts of research centers. Within the Division, the Transfusion Medicine Research Group is active in a number of ongoing projects.

INDEX

Numbers in italics refer to tables or figures

A

Absolute risk, 96-97
Adverse outcomes, risk of, 10, 97-98
Allocation bias, 7, 39
Allogeneic red cells
    infectious disease markers in, 71
    reducing use, 92-93
Alloyed standard, 16
Analytic studies, 2-3
Antibody identification, 72-73, 78
Ascertainment bias, 39
Associate editors, 138, 141-145
Assumptions in statistical testing
    confounding variables, absence of, 66-68
    data collection, 73-74
    generalizability, 69-71
    in mathematical models, 72-73
    measurements, repeat, 71-72
    publication of statistical tests, 74
    randomization, 68-69
    statistical tests, specified, 72-73
Audits, transfusion, 70
Authors' instructions, 140, 142
Autologous blood
    and hemoglobin levels, 69-70
    infectious disease markers in, 71
    methods of recovery study, 92-93
Average effect, 31
Awards
    career development, 165-167
    minority programs, 168-170
    National Research Service, 167-168
    See also Grants

B

Baseline variables, 89-92
Bayes' theorem, 84-86
Bayesian statistical analysis, 86-87
Belmont Report, 107-108
Beneficence, 107
Bias
    in control groups, 8-9
    in data collection, 23, 73-74
    definition, 39
    observation (ascertainment), 39
    publication, 65-66, 74
    in randomization, 7-8, 46, 68-69
    in results, 4, 6, 24
    selection (allocation), 7, 39
    in test evaluations, 16
Blinded studies, 9, 46, 50, 51
Blocked randomization, 68-69
Blood Resources Program, 151, 156-157

C

Career development grants, 165-167
Case-control/referent studies, 5
    See also Retrospective studies
Catheters, indwelling urinary, and postoperative UTI, 40, 42
Centers. *See* Research Centers
Chimpanzees, 161
CI. *See* Confidence intervals
Clinical trials
    blinded studies, 9
    control groups, 8-9
    data collection, 22-23

ethical issues, 24-25
goals, 9
protocol, written, 20-21
randomization in, 7-9
results, analysis, 24
selection of study populations, 7-9, 21-22
study types, 6-7
See also Randomized controlled trials
CMV. *See* Cytomegalovirus
Cohort studies, 18-19
See also Prospective studies
Coinvestigators, 134-135
Collaborative research, 127
Comparison groups. *See* Control groups
Confidence intervals, 24, 81, 87-88
Confidentiality, 114-115, 119-120
Conflict of interest, 136-137, 141
Confounding factors/variables
definition, 39, 67
effects on statistical testing, 66-68
and exaggerated treatment effects, 51
minimizing with sample size, 46-47
in observational studies, 39-45
reducing with randomization, 43-44, 68-69, 89-92
Consultants, 134-135
Contingency tables, 36, 44-45
Contracts
Request for Proposals, 153-154, *155*
research projects, active, 159-161
Control groups, 8-9, 22
Cooperative agreements, 153-154, *155*
Copy editor, 145-146
Cord blood banking, 127-129, 160-161
Cord Blood Stem Cell Transplantation Study, 160-161
Criterion standard, 16
Cross-sectional studies, 5-6, 12, 18
Cutoff point value of tests, 15-16
Cytomegalovirus, and filtered blood, 70-71, 82-83

D

Data
bias in, 23, 73-74
hard (objective), 22-23
paired, 94-96
presentation using descriptive statistics, 92-98
soft (subjective), 22-23
Data analysis in study designs, 24, 134
See also Meta-analysis
Data collection, 22-23, 73-74
Data dredging, 72, 73
Declaration of Helsinki, 107
Department of Health and Human Services
qualifications of research studies, 109-110
regulations, human subjects research, 108-109
Descriptive statistics
absolute *vs* relative risk, 96-97
adverse outcomes, risk of, 97-98
distribution of data, 92-94
in paired data, 94-96
Descriptive studies, 2-3
Device determination, 126-127
DHHS. *See* Department of Health and Human Services
Diagnostic tests. *See* Tests
Disease monitoring. *See* Surveillance systems
Disease prevalence
and statistical tests, 84-86
in surveillance, 18-19
use in screening tests, *14*, 15
Division of Blood Diseases and Resources of the NHLBI
budget analysis, 154-157
programs, 150-151
Transfusion Medicine Group projects, 157-161
Double-blind studies, 9, 51

E

Editors, 138, 141-146
Efficacy of treatments, 9, 10
Epidemiologic studies, 9-12

Equivalence, 81-83
Ethical issues
    in clinical trials, 25
    communication of results to subjects, 115
    confidentiality, 114-115
    future testing, 115-116
    history of, 106-107
    and IRB reviews, 110
    linkage, 114
    progenitor and cord blood banking, 127-129
    and study designs, 122-124
Evaluation of therapies and procedures, 6-12
Expedited reviews, 112-113, 126-127
Experimental studies, 3, 7-9
Exposure status, 2-6

F

False-positive/negative test results, 13, 17
FDA. *See* Food and Drug Administration
Filters, blood and CMV, 70-71, 82-83
Fixed-effects method, 36, 37
Follow-up studies. *See* Prospective studies
Food and Drug Administration, regulations, human subjects research, 108-111
Forms
    data collection, 22
    informed consent, 117-121
Funding, research
    contracts, 159-161
    Division of Blood Diseases and Resources, 154-157
    grants, 157-159, 161-167
    investigator-initiated, 151-152
    listing sources, 141
    minority programs, 168-170
    National Research Service Awards, 167-168
    NHLBI-initiated, 152-154

G

Galley review, 146
Generalizability, 69-71
Gold standard, 16
Grants
    FIRST awards, change in policy, 164-165
    mechanisms, 161-165
    Request for Applications, 153-156
    research career development, 165-167
    Research Center, 165
    research projects, active, 157-159
    See also Awards

H

Hard (objective) data, 22-23
HCV. *See* Hepatitis C
Hemoglobin levels, and preoperative autologous donations, 69-70, 94-95
Hemoglobin-based oxygen carriers, 158
Hepatitis C
    posttransfusion, natural history, 159
    use of chimpanzees in research, 161
Heterogeneity of effects, *38*
HIV in current research, 158-159, 160, 161
Homogeneity of effects, 37
Human subjects research
    collaborative research, 127
    communication of results to subjects, 115
    confidentiality, 114-115
    consent for future testing, 115-116
    device determinations, 126-127
    ethical issues, 24-25, 106-107, 110
    expedited review, 112-113, 126-127
    informed consent, 116-122
    IRB review and approval, 109-113, 122-124, 136
    linkage, 114
    with materials or data collected for tranfusions, 124-125

progenitor and cord blood banking, 127-129
recruitment of subjects, 116
regulations, 105-109
repositories, 125-126
and risk levels, 111-112
source materials, origin of, 116
study designs, impact of regulations on, 113-116
Hypothesis testing, 81

I

Infection, postoperative, and allogenic blood transfusion, 36-41, 44-45, 48-52
Infectious disease testing, 71
Information, collecting. *See* Data collection
Informed consent
administration, 116, 122
for future testing, 115-116
and IRB reviews, 123
progenitor and cord blood banking, 127-129
in study design, 25
waiver of, 115, 117, 124-125, 128
written forms, 117-121
Institutional Review Board
approval required by journals, 136
exemptions from review, 110-111
expedited review, 112-113
facilitating review process, 122-124
human subjects research, 124-129
impact on study design, 113-116
informed consent, 117-122
mission, 109
review and approval criteria, 109-113
waiver of informed consent, 115, 117, 124-125, 128
Intention-to-treat analysis, 51-52
IRB. *See* Institutional Review Board

J

Journals
approval for publication, 144-145
editorial office, 138, 141-142
examples, 138
instructions to authors, 140, 142
production, 145-147
review of manuscript, 142-143, 144
revisions, 143-144
selecting for publication, 139-140
submitting manuscripts, 140-141
See also Publishing
Justice, 107-108

L

Laboratory personnel and procedures, 133
Linkage, 114
Longitudinal studies. *See* Prospective studies

M

Manuscripts
acceptance, 144-145
consideration by journals, 138
formats, 140
production, 145-147
review of, 141-143, 144
revisions, 143-144
submitting, 140-141
See also Journals; Publishing
Mathematical models, 63-64
McNemar's test, 94
Mean, 92-93
Meta-analysis
component parts, 35-39
fixed-effects method, 36, 37
quality of RCTs for inclusion, 46-53
quality scores, using, 48, *50*, 52-53
random-effects method, 37

INDEX 175

RCTs *vs* observational studies, 43-45
restricted to RCTs, 39-45
selection of studies, 52-53
sequence of steps, 33-34
uses, 31, 32-35, 47, 54-55
Minimal risk studies
expedited review, 112-113
in human subject research, 111-113
waiver of informed consent, 117, 124
Minority research awards, 168-170
Monoclonal antibodies, human HIV, 158-159
Multiple pairwise comparisons, 76
Multiple Project Assurance Compliance, 109

N

National Heart, Lung, and Blood Institute (NHLBI)
career development grants, 165-167
current research projects, 157-161
Division of Blood Diseases and Resources, 150-151
funding mechanisms, 154-157
grant mechanisms, 161-165
institute research projects, 152-154
investigator-initiated, 151-152
minority programs, 168-170
mission, 149-150
National Research Service Awards, 167-168
research centers, 165
units, 150
National Research Service Awards (NRSA), 167-168
Negative studies, 24, 80
NHLBI. *See* National Heart, Lung, and Blood Institute
Null hypothesis
determining clinical significance, 88
proving/disproving with p values, 81, 83-87
Nuremberg Code, 107

O

Objective data, 22-23
Observation bias, 39
Observational studies
confounding factors, 39-45
epidemiologic, 9-12
limitations, 39-43
meta-analysis of, *vs* RCTs, 43-45
vs experimental studies, 3
Odds ratio, 36, 44, 45
On-treatment analysis, 52
Outcome data, 3-6
Outcomes, adverse, 97-98

P

p values
comparing baseline variables, 89-92
and confounding variables, 67
in data collection, 72-74
definition, 66
generation of too many, 74-78
limitations, 87-88
and publication bias, 65-66, 74
in repeat measurements, 71-72
and sample size, 79-80
statistically insignificant results between groups, 78-79
statistically significant results between groups, 83-87
using to prove/disprove null hypotheses, 81, 83-87
vs confidence intervals, 87-88
PAD. *See* Preoperative autologous donation
Page proof review, 146
Paired data (studies), 94-96

Paired t test, 94-95
Personnel, laboratory, 133
Pharmacoepidemiology, 10
Phase III studies, 6-9
Phase IV studies, 6, 10
Placebos, 8, 9
Platelets
    trial to reduce alloimmunization to (TRAP), 158
    viability and function post-transfusion, 159
Point estimate, 87
Positive predictive value, 14, 15
Postmarketing surveillance, 10
Power of a statistical test, 85-86
Predictive values, 84-86
Preoperative autologous donation (PAD), 94-95
Prevalence studies. See Cross-sectional studies
Procedures, laboratory, 133
Progenitor cell banking, 127-129
Program announcement (PA), 154
Program project grants, 154, 155
Prospective studies, 4
    eliminating bias, 73-74
    epidemiologic, 11
    surveillance system, 184
Protocol, 125-126
    amendments to, 125-126
    importance of, 26
    review of, 25
    writing, 20-21, 135-136
Publishing
    bias in, 65-66, 74
    of statistical tests, 74
    study planning, 131-137
    types of publications, 137
    See also Journals; Manuscripts

Q

Quality control studies, 110
Quality scores of RCTs, 48, 50, 52-53

R

Random assignment, 7-8, 11
Random-effects method, 37

Randomization
    benefits of, 51-52
    bias in, 7-8, 46, 68-69
    in distribution of baseline variables, 89-92
    methods, 49, 68
    in RCTs, 43-44, 46, 47
    types, 68-69
    See also Randomized controlled trials
Randomized controlled trials
    bias in, 46
    confounding factors, reducing, 43-44
    defined, 43
    limitations of, 47, 49, 51-52
    quality of, 46-53
    quality scores, 48, 50, 52
    sample sizes in, 46-47
    selection of studies, 52-53
    subjects, assignment of, 49, 51
    transfusion and postoperative infection, 36-39
    use in meta-analysis, 32-33, 39-45
    validity of results, 48-52
    vs observational studies, 43-45
    See also Randomization
RCT. See Randomized controlled trials
Receiver-operating characteristic (ROC) curve, 16
Recruitment of subjects, 116
Regulations
    human subjects research, 105-108
    impact on study designs, 113-116
Relative risk, 38, 96-97
Repeat measurements, 71-72
Repository, 125-126, 161
Reprints of manuscripts, 146-147
Request for Applications (RFAs), 153-154, 155
    research projects, active, 157-159
Request for Proposals (RFPs), 153-154

research projects, active, 159-161
Research Centers, *155*, 156, 165
Research initiatives, NHLBI, 152-153
Research projects
    active, 159-161
    collaborative, 127
    conflict of interest, 135-136, 141
    consultants or coinvestigators, 134-135
    funding, 141, 151-157
    grants, 153-167
    human subjects, 105-130
    IRB approval, 105-130
    NHLBI initiatives, 152-153
    p values, importance of, 65-66
    planning, 131-137
    protocol, 20-21, 135-136
    publication of results, 131-147
    purpose for the study, 132, 136
    reasons for the study, 131-132, 135, 136
    skills required, 133-134
    source material needed, 116, 135
    types, 132-133
    See also Study designs; Statistical analysis
Retrospective studies, 4-5
    bias in, 73-74
    epidemiologic, 11-12
    in evaluating diagnostic tests, 13
Retrovirus Epidemiology Donor Study (REDS), 159
RFAs. *See* Request for Applications
RFPs. *See* Request for Proposals
Risks
    absolute *vs* relative, 96-97
    of adverse outcomes, 97-98
    distribution, studies in, 90-92
    minimal, studies, 111-113, 117, 124
    as subjects of studies, 119

ROC curve, 16
RR. *See* Relative risk
Rule of three, 97

S

Safety of treatments, 9, 10
Sample sizes
    effect of p values, 79-80
    minimizing confounding factors, 46-47
    and statistically significant results, 82
SCOR. *See* Specialized Centers of Research
Screening tests. *See* Tests
Selection bias, 39
Sensitivity
    calculations, *14, 15*, 16
    definition, 12
    of diagnostic/screening tests, 12-17
    and statistical tests, 84-86
Septic complications, postoperative, 40, *41*
Sequential statistical testing, 77-78
Simple randomization, 68
Single-blind studies, 9, 46
Skills required for research, 133-134
Soft (subjective) data, 22-23
Solicitation documents
    Program announcement (PA), 154
    Request for Applications (RFAs), 153-154, *155*
    Request for Proposals (RFPs), 153-154
    review of, 153-154
Source material, 116, 135
Specialized Centers of Research (SCOR), 151, 154, 165
Specificity
    calculations, *14, 15*, 16
    defined, 12
    of diagnostic/screening tests, 12-17
    and statistical tests, 84-86
Standard deviation (SD), 92-93
Statistical analysis

assumptions, 66-74
Bayesian, 86-87
descriptive statistics, 92-98
extent needed in research projects, 134
as a mathematical model, 63-65
vs diagnostic tests, 84-86
See also P values
Statistical overview. *See* Meta-analysis
Statistical testing. *See* P values; Statistical analysis
Statistically significant results. *See* P values
Study amendments, 125-126
Study cohorts, 18-19
Study designs
amendments to, 125-126
analytic, 2-3
cross-sectional, 5-6
data collection, 22-23
definition, 1
descriptive, 2-3
diagnostic tests, evaluation of, 12-17
disease monitoring, 17-20
epidemiological, 9-12
ethical issues, 24-25, 122-124
experimental, 3, 7-9
informed consent, 116-122
IRB review process, facilitating, 122-124
observational, 3, 9-12, 39-45
prospective, 4
protocol, 20-21, 135-136
regulations, impact of, 113-116
results, analysis and reporting, 24
retrospective, 4-5
study populations, 21-22
treatments, evaluation of, 6-12
See also Clinical trials; Bias
Study populations
baseline variables, randomization of, 89-92
See also Subject selection
Study sample, 21-22
Subgroup analysis, 76-77

Subject selection
in clinical trials, 7-10, 21-22
in cross-sectional studies, 5-6
informed consent, 118
in prospective studies, 4
in RCTs, 32-33
in retrospective studies, 4-5
in study design, 21-22
Subjective data, 22-23
Subjects, human. *See* Human subjects research
Summary effect, 31
Surveillance systems, 17-20
Surveys. *See* Cross-sectional studies

T

t test, 94-95
Tables, contingency, 36, 44-45
Target population, 21-22
Termination of study, 120
Testing, future, 115-116
Tests, diagnostic or screening
cutoff point values, selecting, 16
detection limit, 13
evaluation, 12-17
positive predictive value, 14
predictive value, 84
purpose, 12, 16-17
sensitivity, 12-17, 84
specificity, 12-17, 84
validity, 12-13
vs statistical tests, 84-86
Tests, statistical
publication of, 74
sequential, 77-78
specification, 72-73
vs diagnostic tests, 84-86
See also Statistical analysis
Therapies. *See* Treatments
Transfusion medicine
audits, 70
confounding variables in, 67-68
equivalency studies in, 82-83
generalizability of studies, 69-71

mathematical models in, 63-64
SCOR program, 157
Transfusion Medicine Scientific Research Group
    funding, 156-157
    grant mechanisms, 161-164
    new investigators policy, 164-165
    request for applications (grants), 157-159
    request for proposals (contracts), 159-161
    research career development grants, 165-167
    research centers, 165
Transfusions, blood
    and infections, postoperative, 36-41, 44-45, 48-52
    platelets, 158-159
    reducing use of, 92-93
    use of filters and CMV, 70-71, 82-83
    and UTI, postoperative, 40, 42
TRAP (Trial to Reduce Alloimmunization to Platelets), 158, 162
Treatment groups, effect of size on p values, 79-80
Treatments
    average or summary effect, 31
    in clinical trials, efficacy, 9, 10
    compared with risk factors, 90-92
    confidence intervals, 81
    efficacy and meta-analysis, 32-33
    equilvalence, 78-83
    evaluation of, 6-12
    exaggerated results in RCTs, 49, 51
    in meta-analysis, 36-38
    random assignment of, 7-8
    to subjects injured in study, 120
    withholding of standard or alternatives, 119
Trials, clinical. *See* Clinical trials
Type II errors, 79

U

Unblinded RCTs, 46, *50*
Urinary tract infections, postoperative, 40, 42
UTI. *see* Urinary tract infections

V

Variables
    baseline, 89-92
    confounding, 39-47, 51, 66-69, 89-92
Virus Activation Transfusion Study (VATS), 160
Viruses
    assays for detection, 160
    blood-borne, 159, 160
    transfusion-transmitted, 158

W

Waiver of informed consent, 115, 117, 124-125, 128
Withdrawal from study, 120-121